LEARN WHAT Q
WHAT KINDS OF T
BE SKEPTICAL, BE SMAR

*WHAT YOUR DOCT(
ABOUT PARKINSON'S DISEASE.*

TRUE OR FALSE:

- Certain workplace and environmental exposures can influence a person's risk of developing the disease. (see page 22)

- Most patients have the motor symptoms of Parkinson's disease for up to five ye_____d. (see page 12)

- The signs and symp_____ilar to those of Parkinson's

- You can consider using alternative therapies early on in the course of your Parkinson's disease in place of medication. (see page 83)

- Your age makes a difference in the medication you should take. (see page 94)

- The longer you have Parkinson's disease, the more likely it is that you will be on multiple medications. (see page 97)

- People with Parkinson's disease should choose organic unsprayed fruits and vegetables, as well as organic grains, dairy products, and meats. (see page 202)

"Dr. Jill Marjama-Lyons is not only an extraordinary physician dedicated to the treatment of Parkinson's disease and other movement disorders, but truly devoted to patient education."
—William C. Koller, M.D., Ph.D., **professor of neurology**

What Your Doctor May *Not* Tell You About

PARKINSON'S DISEASE

A Holistic Program for Optimal Wellness

JILL MARJAMA-LYONS, M.D. and MARY J. SHOMON

WARNER BOOKS

An AOL Time Warner Company

Neither the publisher, nor the authors, nor any of the medical, health, or wellness practitioners or patients quoted in this book take responsibility for any possible consequences from any treatment, procedure, exercise, dietary modification, action, or application of medication or preparation by any person reading or following the information in this book. The publication of this book does not constitute the practice of medicine, and this book does not attempt to replace your physician or your pharmacist. Before you undertake any course of treatment, the author and publisher advise you to consult with your physician or health practitioner regarding any prescription drugs, vitamins, minerals, and food supplements or other treatments and therapies that would be beneficial for your particular health problems and the dosages that would be best for you.

Please note also that while patient stories are real, names have been changed to protect patients' privacy.

Copyright © 2003 by Jill Marjama-Lyons, M.D. and Mary J. Shomon
All rights reserved.

The title of the series What Your Doctor May *Not* Tell You about . . . and the related trade dress are trademarks owned by Warner Books and may not be used without permission.

Warner Books, Inc., 1271 Avenue of the Americas, New York, NY 10020

Visit our Web site at www.twbookmark.com.

An AOL Time Warner Company

Printed in the United States of America

First Printing: February 2003

10 9 8 7 6 5 4 3 2 1

Library of Congress Cataloging-in-Publication Data
Marjama-Lyons, Jill.
    What your doctor may not tell you about Parkinson's disease : a holistic program for optimal wellness / Jill Marjama-Lyons and Mary J. Shomon.
        p. cm.
    Includes bibliographical references and index.
    ISBN 0-446-67890-2
    1. Parkinson's disease—Popular works. 2. Parkinson's disease—Alternative treatment.
I. Shomon, Mary J. II. Title.

RC382 .M369 2003
616.8'33—dc21   2002068959

Book design by Charles S. Sutherland
Cover design by Diane Luger

For Mikela, Lindsay, Bridget, Steve, and Julia

Contents

Acknowledgments

A lot of effort went into the making and writing of this book. I would first like to thank Mary Shomon, my coauthor, for finding me and inviting me to join her in this project, for her writing, and for her guidance and insight. I would also like to thank our agent, Carol Mann, and editor, John Aherne, for this wonderful opportunity and their support. Next, I would like to thank all of my colleagues who gave advice and helped in many of the sections of this book. I am indebted to my mentor, Dr. William Koller, for teaching me so much during my fellowship year and continuing to guide me in my career and for his dedication to research in the field of Parkinson's disease (PD). I am grateful to Dr. Irwin Montgomery for his interest in me as a neurology resident and for his encouragement to pursue the study of Parkinson's disease; Dr. Rajish Pahwa for his editing and friendship and dedication to the study of deep brain stimulation; Dr. Genera Holladay and Joe Nelson for teaching t'ai chi and for their caring manner and holistic treatment of PD patients with acupuncture and herbs; Wanda Barnes, R.N., for teaching yoga at the Jacksonville center; Dr. Matt Farrer,

Director of Neurogenetics at the Mayo Clinic, Jacksonville, for his support of the Florida Society of Movement Disorders and his editing of the genetics sections of this book; Ruth Hagestuen, M.A., R.N., Program Director for the National Parkinson Foundation (NPF), for her editing and commitment to the development of better care for all people with Parkinson's disease; Dr. Abe Lieberman, National Medical Director of NPF, for bringing me to Florida, for his support of my career and of the University of Florida Parkinson Center in Jacksonville as well as the many NPF Centers around the world; Nathan Slewett, Chairman of NPF, and Herbert Zemel, President of NPF, for their undying commitment to the success of the National Parkinson Foundation. I need to thank Jean Barr, R.N., for blessing every patient that has had the privilege to know her caring heart and hands, and my sincere gratitude to Dr. Karen Parko, director of Neurology at Northern Navajo Medical Center, for inviting me into the world of the Dineh. A very special thanks to my dear friend and colleague, Dr. Barbara Maddoux, for her contributions to the mind-body section of this book and for opening my mind and for continuing to educate me in the world of alternative therapies. Thank you to Valerie Bauler and Judy Murakami of Medtronic, Inc., for allowing us to use their pictures depicting deep brain stimulation. I especially want to thank all of my patients throughout my entire training for sharing their stories and for sharing their lives with me and for teaching me more about Parkinson's disease and life than anyone. I would like to thank my parents, Owen and Patricia Marjama, for their emotional support, and especially my mother for her editing and spiritual guidance. And more than anyone, I would like to thank my husband, Mike Lyons, for his help with filing, mailing, and online searches and for his infinite patience and unconditional love and for giving me the most inspirational gift in this world, our children.

—*Jill Marjama-Lyons, M.D.*

First, I'd like to thank Jill Marjama-Lyons, who is everything a physician should be—smart, tireless, innovative, and truly caring. Every Parkinson's disease patient deserves a doctor this incredible, and every writer should be so lucky as to collaborate with such a smart, open-minded and talented coauthor. This book would not be a reality without the remarkable abilities and support of both our agent, Carol Mann, and our editor at Warner, John Aherne. I would also like to thank my husband, Jon Mathis, who helps keep things together so wonderfully when I am knee-deep in working on the latest book. Without his love and support, this book would not have been possible. I also want to thank my daughter Julia, who is always more patient than she should be while Mommy is "making another book." Special thanks to family, friends, and supporters who provided love, support, assistance, patience, and encouragement all along the way, including Dan Shomon, Sr., Pat Shomon, Barbara and Russell Mathis, Jeannie Yamine, Michele Abdow, Angela Cannon, the Momfriends list, Ric and Diane Blake, Elizabeth Mensah-Engmann, Rosario Quintanilla, and Ana Quintanilla. Special thanks go to James Scheer and Marie Savard, M.D., for their research, guidance, input, and valuable information. For top-notch research, writing, Internet consulting, and technical help, I am also very thankful for the assistance of: Kim Conley, Laura Horton, Louise Shapiro, and Vickie Queen.

—*Mary J. Shomon*

◈ CONTRIBUTORS

The authors would like to thank the following contributors for their input, support, and information:

Wanda Barnes, R.N., Certified Kripalu Yoga Instructor, Jacksonville, Florida

Valerie Bauler and Judy Murakami, Medtronic, Inc.

Phylameana lila Desy, holistic healer and Reiki practitioner, Burlington, Iowa

Matt Farrer, Ph.D., Director of Neurogenetics, Mayo Clinic Jacksonville, Jacksonville, Florida

Ruth Hagestuen, M.A., R.N., National Program Director, the National Parkinson Foundation Headquarters, Miami, Florida

Stan Harris, father, minister, friend, and person with Parkinson's

Genera Holladay, Ph.D., Licensed Acupuncturist, herbalist, Registered Pharmacy Consultant, and t'ai chi instructor, Jacksonville, Florida

William Koller, M.D., Ph.D., Director of Parkinson Research, the Parkinson Center, University of Miami, Miami, Florida

Stephen Langer, M.D., holistic physician and author of *Solved: The Riddle of Illness,* Berkeley, California

Barbara Maddoux, R.N., D.O.M. (Doctor of Oriental Medicine), holistic practitioner and licensed yoga instructor, Albuquerque, New Mexico

Joe Nelson, Licensed Acupuncturist, licensed t'ai chi instructor, and martial artist, Jacksonville, Florida

Mary Noone, artist, Glenwood Springs, Colorado

Rajish Pahwa, M.D., Medical Director of the NPF Parkinson Center of Excellence, Kansas University, Kansas City, Kansas

David Perlmutter, M.D., of the Perlmutter Health Center in Naples, Florida, and author of *BrainRecovery.com.*

Marie Savard, M.D., patient advocate and author of *How to Save Your Own Life: The Savard System for Managing—And Controlling—Your Health Care* and *The Savard Health Record: A Six-Step System for Managing Your Healthcare*

Foreword

I will always remember the first time I met Dr. Jill Marjama-Lyons in the ICU at St. Joseph Hospital in Albuquerque. She had left her doctor's bag on the counter outside a room where she was seeing a patient. There was a black and white panda bear sticking out of the top. Curious, I examined the bag more closely and discovered a turtle as well. Tools of the trade for a pediatrician, perhaps, but I knew Jill was a neurologist. I knew then that I had to get to know this woman. She later explained that the turtle energy was important to keep those of us in the health profession grounded, and the panda represented the Oriental energy of the martial arts that she had studied and that had become such an important part of her life. As an intensive care unit nurse, I had found that discussions of this nature were few and far between, except at the yoga studio where I practiced. It was extraordinary to see a physician with such an in-depth understanding of the multifaceted aspects of the human experience that she was able to integrate and weave them into a holistic plan of care. It is that depth and breadth of experience and point of view that make this book such an extraordinary endeavor and truly a labor of love.

Dr. Marjama-Lyons's efforts to bring this information to patients everywhere, not just in her clinic, is commendable. Patients and physicians everywhere will truly benefit from learning the knowledge and concepts of complementary and alternative medicine presented here. By sharing our knowledge and experience, we hope to inspire everyone, patients and physicians alike, to think beyond the realm of what is right before their eyes. This landmark book should be an inspiration to us all to think about our health—not just Parkinson's disease—in ways not before even considered.

—*Barbara Maddoux, R.N., D.O.M.*

Three years ago, at age 43, I was referred to a neurologist who diagnosed me with Parkinson's disease. With four children, and having recently begun my second career, I suddenly found myself faced with a spiraling decline in my ability to provide for my family. Prior to my diagnosis, I had always been in excellent health and had therefore given little attention to my physical well-being, although I did have a casual interest in a holistic approach to health. With the onset of PD and through the encouragement of my wife, I began to learn all I could about complementary medicine, especially as it related to my condition.

It was during this quest for knowledge that I became acquainted with the Parkinson Center at Shands Hospital in Jacksonville, and with Dr. Jill Marjama-Lyons, the Parkinson Center director at that time. My wife made the initial consult visit and came home exclaiming, "They believe in treating the whole person!" From that initial contact, along with attendance at a symposium hosted by the center, I knew that I needed to change doctors—I wanted to see Dr. Marjama-Lyons.

There is no doubt I could have continued with my first neurologist and received competent medical treatment. I hate to think, however, of all that I would have missed out on if I had not become familiar with a team of medical professionals who recognize that quality of life includes more than dopamine in a brain. Those who treat me don't have all the answers, but they are open to all the answers, from wherever they come. Nutrition, exercise, natural supplements, spirituality, various European and Oriental treatments—they all play a part, not to the exclusion of traditional medicine, but incorporated with it. As a Parkinson's patient, the greatest benefit that comes from a holistic approach to my treatment is the support that I feel from a team of people who don't blindly follow the suggestions of political correctness, but rather, who do what is right for me, the patient.

I would encourage other Parkinson's patients to find a doctor whom you trust and who will trust you. Discuss your interest, plans, and understanding about holistic therapies. We each need to take an active role in our own treatment, but we also need a professional to manage that treatment. I recommend this book for all who are associated with Parkinson's disease in any way: patient, caregiver, and professional. I recommend it to those Parkinson's disease patients interested in improving their health in general, and to those who are in the business of improving health. Lastly, I recommend it to the skeptic who will take time to read a few of these pages with an open mind.

—Stan Harris, Parkinson's disease patient

Introduction

When East meets West
When the desert meets the sea
When doctor becomes patient
When white woman meets red man
Then we will begin to walk on the path to understanding
    —*The Path to Understanding,* by Jill Marjama-Lyons

More than a million Americans have Parkinson's disease. It's a disease that affects many people of different races and cultures, men and women, young and old. It can be disabling in a variety of ways, but primarily affects patients by causing difficulty with motor function. People with Parkinson's disease may struggle with simple tasks such as getting out of bed, buttoning a shirt, or walking from the bedroom to the kitchen. They may be embarrassed by a hand that trembles or have trouble with their balance.

Ultimately, living well with Parkinson's disease requires knowledge—knowledge of how Parkinson's affects both mind and body, knowledge of traditional Western medicine and complementary and holistic therapies that can aid in treatment.

In *What Your Doctor May Not Tell You about Parkinson's*

Disease, you'll find a book that provides that knowledge. This book will help you if . . .

- You strongly suspect you have Parkinson's disease, but are having difficulty getting a diagnosis.
- You aren't sure whether your symptoms point to Parkinson's and you want to find out more.
- You have been diagnosed with Parkinson's disease, and all you were told was to take your medicine and come back in a year.
- You are being treated for Parkinson's disease, but you don't feel well, you don't think your treatment is making a difference, and you want something better.
- You are interested in complementary/alternative approaches to treating your Parkinson's disease symptoms.
- You are a health care provider and are interested in a holistic approach to the treatment of your patients with Parkinson's disease by combining traditional and nontraditional therapies.
- You are the spouse or family member of a person with Parkinson's disease and want to know more about what to expect, and how to help your Parkinson's patient.

Above all, this book is for you if you want to learn how to achieve optimal physical and spiritual health with Parkinson's disease from the perspective of empowering patients, families, and caring health practitioners.

In this book, you'll find out what your doctor may not tell you about risk factors, diagnosis, drugs, surgery, and alternative and conventional things that work—and don't work—to treat Parkinson's disease. You'll also hear the voices of patients and their spouses, real people who have struggled for a diagnosis, learned to deal with doctors, tried different medications, used alternative therapies, had brain surgery, suffered setbacks, and enjoyed successes. Each person quoted in this book shares his or her own story, thoughts, fears, and hopes with you. You will recognize your own similar experiences, thoughts, and emotions in the honest and poignant stories from patients of all backgrounds. Most important, you will know that you are not alone.

This book will help you learn what questions to ask, what kinds of doctors and health care providers to seek, and what types of therapies you might want to pursue. Of course, each person is completely different and deserves and needs an individualized treatment plan. But this book will help you be an educated self-advocate. You'll learn how to find doctors and practitioners who will help you create the right program— with whatever conventional and alternative approaches work for you.

You'll also learn that, whether it's the word of a doctor, practitioner, or even what you read in this book, you should not blindly accept what anyone tells you about your health. By "anyone" I mean just that, including your medical doctors with their many diplomas, your nurses, licensed therapists of all backgrounds, your family and friends, and even yourself.

Ultimately, the right path will resonate within your soul, heart, and mind. Be skeptical, be smart, be patient, and know that living with a long-term physical illness will be an evolving, dynamic process. You can grow in your understanding not only of how to cope, but also of how to survive and even flourish and go beyond what others have told you you can do. Let yourself be open to all sorts of options, traditional and nontraditional, for treating your illness and enhancing the health and wellness of your mind, body, and spirit.

◈ SPIRIT

Before I began writing this book, I meditated and I prayed for guidance. I wanted this book to be helpful to those who read it, something that would hopefully make a positive difference, even if in a small way. And the message I received was very clear—spirituality had to penetrate and permeate this book. It had to be found in every chapter, on every page, and in every word.

Parkinson's disease is a physical illness that causes difficulty with motor function. So much of the emphasis on treating a person with Parkinson's disease is on the physical symptoms—the tremor, muscle slowness, and rigidity—and little, if any, emphasis is put on the emotional, mental, and spiritual health of the patient. In fact, this is true with most physical illnesses, under the Western or traditional medicine approach. We wait until a physical symptom occurs and then attempt to fix it in some way. As doctors, we spend little time in medical school or residency learning about preventative medicine or health—rather, we focus on the disease state.

Parkinson's disease does affect motor function, but it does not take away your spirit, unless you let it. Don't let yourself or the people in your life, even your physician, take your spirit away. No matter what the state of our physical world or health, if we do not attend to our spiritual nature and selves, we cannot truly achieve good health and wellness.

By spirituality, I do not mean religion. I mean our mental, emotional, and nonphysical selves. Without positive thoughts and emotions, without dreams and desires, without faith, hope, love, and spirit, we are nothing. All people die, but very few really learn to live. Learn to live positively with optimal physical and spiritual health whether you have Parkinson's disease or not.

◈ THE JOURNEY INTO MEDICINE AND BEYOND

I knew I wanted to be a doctor in tenth grade. It was a combination of having a crush on my biology teacher, Mr. DuPre, and the pure excitement I felt holding the spinal cord of a moose, and seeing all the organs inside of a dead frog. I was hooked!

I knew I was capable enough to be a doctor and could accomplish anything I wanted to, thanks to my parents and the self-confidence that they instilled in me. They also planted a seed long before the tenth grade. When I was nine years old, they told me to ask Santa for a stethoscope—not a toy, but the real kind that doctors use. So being the obedient, semi-precocious child that I was, I asked and the real stethoscope arrived on schedule on Christmas morning. I took that stethoscope everywhere I went . . . in fact, it is hanging in my closet as I write this on my home computer. While at the University of North Carolina for my undergraduate schooling, when no one else was around, I would put it on around the collar of my lab coat and smile at myself in the mirror of my dorm room, saying, "You look just like a doctor!" So the seed was planted and now the little tree needed to grow.

I grew a little at Chapel Hill, where I learned about psychology and the basic sciences and discovered that the human body and mind fascinated me enough to pursue medical school. I was led back to my home state of New York, back to the snow and downhill skiing, back to the Finger Lakes and bass fishing, back to the fast-paced Northeast and cold, cloudy Syracuse. There, during my first semester of medical school, I found the love of anatomy and the love of my first patient—my cadaver. My cadaver taught me about the brain and all the nerves and their connections to one another. I learned about all the organ systems, the heart, the kidney, liver, lung, and muscles. I learned about the human body, but I also learned about the human spirit. My cadaver had a soul and was once a living being who lived an entire lifetime, and now he lay still, soaked in formaldehyde, here to teach me. Out of death came life—the birth of a physician—plus the basic knowledge of anatomy and the thrill of beginning the journey into medicine.

I worked hard and struggled through four years of medical school and managed to climb from the bottom to the top third of my class. While in the third year of medical school, I had a brief, two-week exposure to neurology, not enough to forge my decision or to draw me into the field. Then, in the fall of my fourth year of medical school, I chose an elective in neurology at the Guthrie Clinic in Sayre, Pennsylvania. During the first week of the rotation, a colleague and I went to examine a patient. We did a diligent history and physical and then went to read and think about our patient before teaching rounds. We deduced that he probably had ALS, amyotrophic lateral sclerosis, also known as Lou Gehrig's disease. On teaching rounds, the attending—the senior neurologist—agreed with our diagnosis and we were delighted. What happened next shocked and horrified me. The attending brusquely told the patient that he had ALS. "You have six more months to live," he said, and then walked out of the room. The intern sheepishly followed, as she was obligated to continue presenting patients to her boss, Dr. No-Bedside-Manner. My feet were frozen; I literally couldn't move. The patient, who was alone—his wife a good two hours' drive away—asked me in his quiet, hoarse voice, "What does that mean, ALS?" I tried to answer with the knowledge I had in as simple lay terms as I could and told him that some people could live many years with this illness, even up to thirteen years, and that we would have to help him with his muscle weakness and his swallowing. In short, I tried to remove the death sentence the attending had just given him and to comfort him as best I could.

It was at that exact moment that I decided to become a neurologist. The defining event was the emotion, the pure anger and outrage at anyone who could be so callous and so coldhearted as to speak to a seriously ill person that way. I decided I needed to become a neurologist, because these patients needed someone who cared and wanted to say the right words in the right way and take the time that needed to be taken to help them cope with a serious and frightening illness.

So, after a year of internship and then a year of psychiatry, I went to the desert, to the red rock mountains and the most beautiful sunsets I had ever seen, to the saguaro cacti and coyote calls at night, to the University of Arizona to learn and study the art of neurology. While in my second year of residency, I saw several patients with Dr. Irwin Montgomery, a Parkinson's specialist and the attending in our department. I was struck by the warm nature and pleasant personalities of the patients I met and was equally in awe of how much better the patients would get when Dr. Montgomery adjusted their medicines. Neurology was often criticized as a field of only diagnosis without effective treatments, and here was a serious neurodegenerative disorder that clearly had very good treatments that made a real difference.

Later that same year, I met a man from Kansas City who invited me to come visit his Parkinson center sometime the next year, so I did and I stayed. There, I had the pleasure of training with Dr. William Koller, an internationally respected expert in the field. And it was there that I fell in love with the wonderful world of Parkinson's disease. A world where delightful people open their hearts and share themselves and their stories as their bodies slow a little and shake a little, a world where positive words and good medicines and surgery make things better, a world of hope of help and healing.

After completing my fellowship in Parkinson's disease, I willingly returned to the high desert and the charm of the Southwest to practice neurology in Albuquerque, New Mexico. The allure of the snow-covered Sandia Mountains in winter and the cool summer night breezes along with the dynamic mixed culture of Native Americans, Hispanics, and Anglos was simply too much to resist. I was surprised at first by the large number of patients that practiced holistic medicine; many of my patients with Parkinson's disease took herbs, saw acupuncturists and massage therapists, and were interested in nutrition and antioxidant therapy. The first year there I met Barbara Maddoux, an intensive care unit nurse then, now Dr. Barbara Maddoux, D.O.M. (Doctor of Oriental Medicine). Her interest in and knowledge of holistic medicine, combined with my patients' experiences, sparked my curiosity and further opened my mind to the real potentials of alternative therapies for the treatment of Parkinson's disease.

My curiosity led me to take up an interest in karate, where I met Mike, the man who would become my husband. Mike and I married, and we soon had two daughters to add to Mike's two children from a previous marriage. During this busy time, I also voluntarily began teaching the neurology residents at the Veteran's Hospital once a month, and that experience rekindled my love of teaching and the academic environment.

I then decided to leave private practice and pursue academic medicine in order to study and learn more about what causes Parkinson's disease, but perhaps more important, to discover and prove what treatments work in the conventional and alternative worlds of medicine. So we packed up the Ford Explorer with the two German shepherds and the minivan with the two babies and our trustworthy nanny, Judy, and drove to Jacksonville, Florida.

The little seed has grown into a tree, a medium-sized aspen with a nice view of the mountains. It is still growing and much of the journey is yet to unfold.

Beyond

There is strength in silence
There is strength in patience
There is strength in wisdom
There is strength in peace
There is strength in unconditional love
There is strength in going beyond the convention and resisting the temptation to blindly follow what they say you must do
There is strength in following your heart and the guidance of God for what you know is true
There is strength in all these things for they are the very things that bond us to one another and set us free
And with them there is great strength in you and me

—Jill Marjama-Lyons, M.D.
www.docjill.com

WHAT YOUR DOCTOR
MAY *NOT* TELL YOU
ABOUT

PARKINSON'S
DISEASE

I am a slow walker, but I never walk backwards.
—*Abraham Lincoln*

Part I

SIGNS, SYMPTOMS, AND DIAGNOSIS

Chapter 1

What Is Parkinson's Disease?

Parkinson's disease cannot take away your hope . . . or your relationships . . . or your dreams . . . or your faith. Parkinson's disease cannot take away your spirit.

—*Jill Marjama-Lyons*

Parkinson's disease was first described in 1817 by James Parkinson, and the disease is named after him. In his classic essay *The Shaking Palsy*, he described the three most prominent features of Parkinson's disease:

- *Tremor*, a rhythmic shaking of a part of the body such as the arm, leg, or chin;
- *Rigidity*, an increase in muscle tone or muscle stiffness; and
- *Bradykinesia*, slowness of movement—for example, walking, writing, or getting out of a chair.

While the actual mechanism behind the disease wasn't understood by Parkinson, experts today understand that Parkinson's disease occurs when a group of cells deep in the middle of the brain—in an area called the substantia nigra compacta (SNc)—begin to malfunction and eventually die. These brain cells, known as neurons, contain a chemical called dopamine, and can be easily seen through a microscope on postmortem examination of the brain. (See figure 1.) The tremor, rigidity, and bradykinesia associated with Parkinson's disease usually become evident after 60 to 70 percent of these dopamine-producing neurons have died.

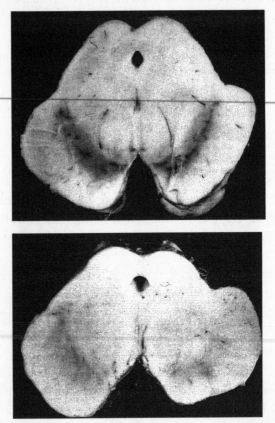

Figure 1. A normal healthy brain (top) and the brain of a person with Alzheimer's disease. The pigmented, dopamine-containing cells of the substantia nigra compacta (SNc) (indicated by the thin dark line) die off, and an Alzheimer's sufferer may lose 50 percent or more of these cells.

❖ THE CAUSES OF PARKINSON'S DISEASE

What causes Parkinson's disease and triggers the neurons to malfunction and die? Scientists have no definitive answers, but many researchers and Parkinson specialists believe that the disease is caused by a number of factors and that it's likely that an environmental factor such as a virus, a toxin, or stress to the body triggers the expression of a genetic, inherited risk in the form of Parkinson's disease. This is called the "double hit" hypothesis, meaning that more than one thing has to occur for a person to get Parkinson's disease.

Oxidative Stress and Free Radicals

Oxidative stress refers to stress on a cell that makes the cell less able to function in its assigned way. Oxidative stress occurs when a cell has become fragmented due to the presence of free radicals. Free radicals are molecules in the body that have become split as a result of various stressors, and that then can attach themselves to other cells or membranes, or even break up other molecules. When free radicals are built up in excessive amounts, they can lead to injury of the cells' proteins and molecules, including DNA, and cause cell death. Oxidative stress is one of the leading theories as to what might cause dopamine cell death in Parkinson's disease.

The body's immune cells can scavenge free radicals, but if the immune system isn't functioning optimally, free radicals can proliferate. The effects of free radicals can be reversed by nutrients known as antioxidants—vitamins C and E are two very common antioxidants, for example. These nutrients are able to give up parts of their cells, which then partner with the free radical and neutralize its destructive capacity.

In the case of Parkinson's disease, researchers are trying to identify those factors that cause oxidative stress on dopamine brain cells. When dopamine is broken down, it is metabolized into several different molecules, including peroxides, which react with iron and form toxic free radicals.

In a healthy brain these peroxides are detoxified by the presence of glutathione. But in a brain where excessive dopamine has caused overproduction of peroxides, or where there is a deficiency of glutathione, overproduction of toxic free radicals can occur and cause oxidative stress and subsequent cell injury and death. Ultimately, when enough cells die, Parkinson's disease symptoms appear. The theory of oxidative stress as a cause of Parkinson's disease is the basis for studies of agents that prevent or lessen oxidative stress, such as glutathione.

Mitochondria, Complex I, NADH, and Coenzyme Q10

The mitochondria are the energy producers of each living cell and are vital for normal cell function. After reports in 1983 that a street drug, MPTP, could cause an acute parkinsonian syndrome in young people who injected the drug intravenously, mitochondria were given center stage as a possible link to the cause of Parkinson's disease. When it enters the body, MPTP is metabolized into MPP+, which is toxic to and causes death of dopamine brain cells. MPP+ does this by entering the mitochondria and interfering with complex I, which is part of the necessary energy-producing machinery of the mitochondria. Specifically, MPP+ inhibits NADH (nicotinamide adenine dinucleotide hydrogen), which blocks the formation of ATP (adenosine triphosphate), the key energy molecule of all cells. When there is no energy for cell function, the result is rapid cell death.

Another important molecule that is part of complex I is Coenzyme Q10 (CoQ10 for short), also called ubiquinone. CoQ10 acts as an antioxidant by binding toxic free radicals, preventing them from killing healthy cells. In fact, this observation led scientists Dr. Richard Haas and Cliff Shults from the University of California, San Diego, to study and show a deficiency or lower activity of CoQ10 in persons with Parkinson's disease. Their research led to a multi-center, National Institutes of Health study of CoQ10 for the treatment of Parkinson's disease, the results of which are expected to shed light on the role of this supplement.

Experts believe that the mitochondria and impaired complex I function appear to have a likely role in the cause of Parkinson's disease and are also looking at other agents that can, like MPP+, interfere with complex I activity. These agents include the pesticide rotenone, diphenylether herbicides, carbon monoxide, hydrogen sulfide, cyanide, and nitric oxide, among others.

Other Theories

Other theories about the causes of Parkinson's disease are covered in chapter 11's discussion of future directions. Some of these cutting-edge ideas—including excitotoxicity, inflammation, apoptosis, and clumping of cellular proteins—may hold keys to the answer of the cause of Parkinson's disease.

❖ UNDERSTANDING PARKINSON'S DISEASE

It is important to have a basic overview of the part of the brain that is affected in Parkinson's disease, to better understand how current medication and surgical therapies work and how future neuroprotective, restorative, and curative treatments will be employed.

Parkinson's Disease's Effects on the Brain

In the brain, nuclei or groups of brain cells (from the substantia nigra, striatum, globus pallidus, subthalamic nucleus, and thalamus) connect to one another and to the part of the brain that controls motor function, the motor cortex. In order for normal movement of the arms and legs to occur, a series of electrical circuits must be fired in a specific pattern and frequency between all of these parts of the brain or nuclei. When one part of this system malfunctions, as it does in Parkinson's disease, then the entire system is affected. In Parkinson's disease, it's the substantia nigra compacta (SNc) that appears to malfunction. The end result of the loss of dopamine cells in the SNc is inhibition or dampening of the electrical signals to the motor cortex.

This part of the brain has so many connections—with motor, sensation, and thinking functions and even the brain stem—that it's thought that the many varied presentations of Parkinson's disease and the many motor and cognitive symptoms of the disease are the result of damage to the various connections. While the mechanism is not truly understood, this damage to the brain's circuitry results in motor symptoms of Parkinson's disease such as bradykinesia, tremors, and rigidity. Medications and surgical treatments available today attempt to restore normal dopamine activity and function of this motor circuit to allow return of normal motor skills.

The Lewy Body

The Lewy body (see figure 2) is a clump of proteins that can be found within the cytoplasm of certain brain cells, typically in people with Parkinson's disease. Lewy bodies are not normally found in brain cells, although rarely they may be seen in small numbers in the brain of an elderly person who has not been diagnosed with Parkinson's disease. There is also a rare disorder, Diffuse Lewy Body Disease, where Lewy bodies are widespread throughout the brain. But the presence of Lewy bodies, when they are primarily found in dopamine cells in the SNc, is considered diagnostic of Parkinson's disease.

The proteins that make up the core of the Lewy body are alpha-synuclein and ubiquitin ligase. These proteins are important in normal cellular function. Ubiquitin ligase is an important enzyme that breaks down abnormally large proteins similar to a garbage disposal, and alpha-synuclein appears to be

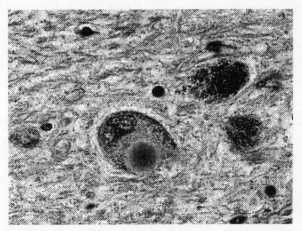

Figure 2. The cell in the center is a Lewy body found in persons with Alzheimer's; a normal dopamine cell, indicated by the darker cluster, is pictured at upper right.

important in the normal folding of cell proteins. Hence abnormal functioning of these proteins may lead to abnormal folding and clumping of proteins and subsequent cell death. It is not known whether the Lewy body is a by-product of cell death or whether it might cause cell death, but researchers agree that the more we learn about the Lewy body, the more we will learn about what causes Parkinson's disease.

Dopamine in Parkinson's Disease

In the normal adult brain there are 400,000 dopamine neurons in the SNc. The dopamine neurons in the SNc release dopamine to stimulate dopamine receptors on nerves in the motor pathway. Dopamine is made by a series of biochemical steps and is also degraded by two main enzymes, MAO and COMT. After 60 to 70 percent of these cells are lost, the motor symptoms of Parkinson's disease develop. As the dopaminergic neurons continue to die off, the motor symptoms gradually and slowly worsen over years. The medications used to treat Parkinson's disease may be dopamine (carbidopa/levodopa is a precursor to dopamine, meaning it is converted by enzymes into dopamine), look like dopamine (dopamine agonists), or act on the enzymes that metabolize dopamine (MAO and COMT inhibitors). So the key to Parkinson's treatment is to restore dopamine activity to normal levels through medications, or through surgery to help restore the brain's electrical signal processing. These treatments are discussed in detail in chapters 5 and 6.

❖ THE PREVALENCE OF PARKINSON'S DISEASE

The *incidence* of a disease is defined as the number of new cases of a disorder diagnosed during a specific period, such as a year, in a defined population, such as people living in a specific geographic region or of a specific race. The *prevalence* of a disease is defined as the total number of persons with the disease at a fixed point in time. Prevalence is easier to measure than incidence, and both are used to report the frequency of a disease and to study and identify risk factors for that illness.

In the United States, over one million people are estimated to have Parkinson's disease. The prevalence is estimated to be as high as 1 in 100 persons over 60 years of age. The median age of onset of Parkinson's disease is between 55 and 60 years, and 10 to 15 percent of patients are diagnosed before age 40, which is considered young-onset Parkinson's disease. The disease is not necessarily a disease of the elderly, but because it is a progressive illness that is more common in older people, as the population itself ages, the number of persons with Parkinson's disease is on the rise. Parkinson's disease affects both men and women, but tends to be slightly more common in men. All cultures and races appear to be affected by Parkinson's disease; however the exact incidence and prevalence among cultures varies somewhat.

❖ THE STAGES OF PARKINSON'S DISEASE

Parkinson's disease is a slowly progressive illness. That means it tends to worsen over many years—ten to thirty—so that the person who has Parkinson's disease will over time notice more difficulty with motor function, such as increasing tremors, more difficulty with fine motor coordination, walking and balance, and possibly more muscle stiffness. Not everyone progresses at the same rate, but in general, the disease progresses slowly, meaning that a person with Parkinson's does not rapidly decline in his or her motor function.

The symptoms usually start on one side of the body (either left or right) and over the course of many years will usually begin to affect the other side. Many patients may have had minor symptoms for five to ten years before being diagnosed. While the fact that the disease is progressive is daunting, the good news is that as the motor symptoms become more pronounced, the currently available treatments—such as medications, surgical procedures, and alternative therapies—can dramatically improve these symptoms. It is imperative to understand that the proper treatment of Parkinson's disease should be a dynamic and ongoing process that will require frequent visits to a Parkinson specialist and other health care providers and will involve periodic adjustments of medications as well as other therapies, such as nutrition, exercise, physical therapy, occupational therapy, speech therapy, massage, and possibly neurosurgery.

There are five stages of Parkinson's disease that have been defined and are outlined below. These definitions are used primarily by Parkinson specialists, often for selecting and following patients that are involved in clinical studies on Parkinson's disease.

It is important to realize that most people who are being treated properly do not progress to Stage IV and very rarely do people progress to Stage V. In addition, a person with Parkinson's disease may have symptoms and a physical examination that, early in the day, before the medication has taken effect, may define his or her status as Stage III, but after the medicine starts working, the patient's status may jump down to Stage II, so the stage can vary within hours or over the course of a day. Persons with Parkinson's disease who are undertreated or improperly treated can enjoy significant improvement with proper therapy, especially with medications and surgery. Some practitioners report seeing patients go from a Stage IV or V without medication down to Stage II or III after being put on correct medicine. This means that people who could not walk without assistance and needed help with virtually everything, such as dressing, feeding, and bathing, can, within several weeks of starting proper medication, walk again and take care of themselves without help.

The Stages of Parkinson's Disease (Modified Hoehn and Yahr Staging)

Stage 0   No signs of disease

Stage I   Unilateral disease (affecting either the left or right side of the body)

Stage I.5   Unilateral disease and axial (neck and back/trunk)

Stage II   Mild bilateral (left and right) disease, without impairment of balance

Stage II.5   Mild bilateral disease, with some mild imbalance

Stage III   Mild to moderate bilateral disease with some difficulty with balance, still physically independent

Stage IV   Moderate to severe bilateral disease with marked disability (needs help with most motor daily tasks such as dressing, bathing, eating), still able to walk or stand without a person assisting, but may need a cane or walker

Stage V   Advanced disease, wheelchair bound or bedridden unless fully aided by another person

◆ A HOLISTIC PERSPECTIVE

In the Traditional Chinese Medicine (TCM) view, Parkinson's disease, as with all diseases, is not identified as a specific condition, but rather matches up to several different constellations of symptoms, each with its own treatment protocol to address the imbalances and deficiencies that are causing that particular group of symptoms. Therefore, someone conventionally diagnosed as having Parkinson's disease whose main symptom was a great deal of tremor could have a very different "diagnosis" in TCM than a Parkinson's patient whose main difficulty was in walking and balance.

Fundamentally, TCM looks at Parkinson's disease as being caused by three categories of symptoms, each signaling that fluids and blood are deficient and are not sufficiently nourishing sinews and energy channels. "Qi and Blood Deficiency" is caused by emotional stress, anger, frustration, and resentment. "Phlegm-Fire Agitating Wind," another category, is thought to be due to diet, in particular, consumption of too much greasy, fried, or sweet foods. A third category consistent with Parkinson's is "Kidney and Liver Yin Deficiency," which is usually due to overwork and insufficient rest, and night or graveyard shifts, which unbalance the body's natural rhythm. TCM then works, using nutrition, herbal remedies, acupuncture, and other TCM approaches, to provide the nutrients and rebalance the movement of energy—qi—to resolve the symptoms.

Complementary and alternative medicine has many different perspectives on Parkinson's disease, but many practitioners view Parkinson's disease as a condition that results from overexposure to toxins, chronic inflammation in the body, insufficient nutrition to the brain, unbalanced blood sugar, and nutritional deficiencies. Using various modalities, including herbs, vitamins, diet, and mind-body approaches, practitioners guide patients in programs that typically consist of several components, including

- Eliminating toxic exposures;
- Avoiding food allergens;
- Ridding the body of pathogens and infectious organisms;
- Providing adequate nutrition and energy to the brain and cells; and
- Introducing anti-inflammatory, detoxifying, and antioxidant foods and supplements.

A detailed look at alternative and complementary medicine, as well as nutritional approaches to Parkinson's disease, is featured in chapters 7 and 8.

Note from Dr. Jill: You Are Not Your Disease!

Before we continue, I want to bring up another important point about what Parkinson's disease is: Parkinson's disease is *not* you, and you are *not* your Parkinson's disease.

I so often hear patients take ownership of their Parkinson's disease by saying, "My Parkinson's disease is acting up or bothering me." How often I have heard doctors and nurses refer to people with Parkinson's disease as "Parkies." I have even caught myself saying, "How's your Parkinson's doing?" rather than saying, "How are you?" Only since working with and treating Navajo people with Parkinson's disease, however, have I come to more fully understand the power of words.

In the Navajo culture, they believe that words are reality, so when I tell a Navajo patient that I think he or she has Parkinson's disease, the words I say are partly responsible for giving the patient Parkinson's disease.

This is an important message. We all have to be careful as doctors, nurses, practitioners, and patients not to define or label others or ourselves by a disease. If we do this, then the disease and its symptoms become our focus. We risk losing the real focus of what we are. We forget that John is an accountant with a wife and children, that he is a man who loves to fish and listen to classical music and has a keen sense of humor, and that he is not a "Parkie." Or that Marie had a career as a professional musician, makes great lasagna, and likes to travel to visit her grandchildren, and is not just "Marie, age 69, diagnosed with Parkinson's in 1995."

So read, find out more about the condition, but do not make the mistake of thinking that you are your disease. Your objective is to learn about the condition and find those therapies and healthy behaviors that work best for you so that you can focus on who you are, rather than on the disease.

I am not saying that you do not have Parkinson's disease, and that it doesn't warrant treatment and adaptation in your life. Rather, if you lead a well-balanced, healthy life by attending to all your needs—physical, emotional, intellectual, and spiritual—and strengthening your connections to others, nature, and the divine, you can achieve optimal wellness and go beyond your disease. You can focus on living well in spite of your illness. You can learn how to cope with and rise above and beyond it, rather than be consumed by it.

J. Kennedy Shultz makes this point in his excellent book *You Are the Power*:

> A consciousness of health is the power that heals. It spends little time thinking about disease or about the excuses for disease, any explanation of disease, any running commentary upon disease. A consciousness of health is entirely focused upon knowing one thing—that health, wholeness of body and being, is our natural state.

Chapter 2

Are You at Risk for Parkinson's Disease?

We know a great deal more about the causes of physical disease than we do about the causes of physical health.

—*M. Scott Peck*

Although the cause of Parkinson's disease is unknown, a number of environmental, toxic, and genetic factors have been linked to the condition. Other factors such as hormone levels and the use of caffeine and nicotine have been proposed as playing a role in the development of Parkinson's disease as well. Ultimately, however, not one single environmental agent has been proven to directly cause Parkinson's disease. And because there has never been an epidemic outbreak of Parkinson's disease, it is unlikely that a single environmental cause exists. Even though several genes have been identified as causes, a purely genetic cause for Parkinson's disease appears to apply to only a very small number of people. The reality is that environmental or toxic exposures, nutritional deficiencies, stressors, and physical and genetic susceptibility combine to trigger Parkinson's disease.

❖ NATURE VERSUS NURTURE?

Scientists in the late 1800s described Parkinson's disease as a purely genetic disorder, and the debate still goes on today regarding whether Parkinson's disease is a genetic (nature) or environmentally derived (nurture) illness. Parkinson's disease was viewed as an inherited disease for some time, until the outbreak of viral encephalitis lethargica—known as sleeping sickness—during World War I. Encephalitis lethargica was described as a slowly progressive parkinsonian syndrome similar to Parkinson's disease.

After this, scientists looked for other possible environmental causes of Parkinson's disease, such as viruses and exposure to heavy metals or toxic chemicals in the workplace. A higher incidence and prevalence of Parkinson's disease was observed with exposure to some of these chemicals and gave credence to the environmental theory. This was even further supported by the discovery that MPTP (a chemically designed synthetic heroin for intravenous drug abusers) induced Parkinson's syndrome in young Northern California IV drug users in the 1980s. However, the compound—MPTP, and its toxic metabolite, MPP+—is not found, except as a designer street drug, in other common chemical sources and cannot account for the large number of persons that develop Parkinson's disease.

In the early 1990s, Dr. Lawrence Golbe described a familial form of Parkinson's disease that affected many members of one very large family of Greek-Italian descent. The gene that caused the disease in this family was then discovered, and the search by geneticists for other genes linked to Parkinson's disease was then reawakened. Several different genes have since been found as causes of the condition, and so the pendulum has begun to swing back toward the genetic theory of Parkinson's disease once again.

❖ RISK FACTOR: GENDER

Parkinson's disease affects both men and women, but the majority of studies have found Parkinson's disease to be slightly more common in men than in women. This trend persists globally, especially in China, where men are three times more likely to get Parkinson's disease than women. Another study found that African, Hispanic, and Caucasian women had a lower incidence of Parkinson's disease than men of the same ethnic groups. One study reported a twofold increase in Parkinson's disease among Italian men across all ages. The explanation for this increased risk in men is not known. It may represent a hormonal effect—estrogen, the primary female hormone, may protect dopamine brain cells from dying. It could also be an environmental/occupational effect, as men are more likely to pursue occupations that expose them to the toxins that are causally linked to Parkinson's disease.

❖ RISK FACTOR: AGE

An increase in age is associated with an increased risk of Parkinson's disease. This has been observed across all cultures and in both sexes. The incidence of Parkinson's disease in one year is less than 10 per 100,000 for persons under the age of 50, compared to over 200 per 100,000 by age 80. It has been estimated that 5 to 10 percent of patients with Parkinson's disease experience the onset of their symptoms before age 40, and the peak incidence of onset of Parkinson's disease is between 55 and 60. Interestingly, the number of persons diagnosed with

Parkinson's disease lessens after age 80, suggesting that the condition is not simply a process due to aging of the brain.

While Parkinson's disease is not necessarily a disease of the elderly, it appears to be on the rise, because as a progressive illness, the risk grows with increased age. So, as the population ages, the number of persons with Parkinson's disease increases.

◈ RISK FACTOR: ETHNICITY

The prevalence of Parkinson's disease appears to vary among races somewhat, and it's thought that there is a higher prevalence in countries where the majority of the population is Caucasian (100 to 300 cases of Parkinson's disease per 100,000 in North America and Europe). The conventional wisdom has also claimed a lower prevalence in Asian and African countries, with 50 cases of Parkinson's disease per 100,000. However, many of these studies are now coming to light as being flawed, and more recent studies have shown a higher prevalence of Parkinson's disease in Americans of African and Asian descent, similar to levels seen in Caucasian Americans. While the prevalence and incidence of Parkinson's disease in Native Americans has not been formally studied, some experts suggest that the prevalence is greater than we originally thought, and may be equal to or even higher than other groups in the American population.

◈ RISK FACTOR: GEOGRAPHIC REGION

The estimated prevalence of Parkinson's disease does vary from region to region. What this means, however, is debatable. For example, 31 per 100,000 persons living in Libya have Parkinson's disease, while the rate is 328 per 100,000 in Bombay,

India. Several studies have shown a difference in the incidence and prevalence of Parkinson's disease in various regions of the United States. These differences could be due to less access to health care, genetic differences in susceptibility to disease, or differences in exposure to causative environmental agents. Even migration patterns can factor into the analysis. If one looks at the state of Florida, for example, with a total population of 16 million, using the standard calculations, 17,600 persons should have Parkinson's disease. However, because Florida is a retirement state, 3.5 million persons are over the age of 60 and the prevalence is therefore even higher, with nearly 40,000 Floridians estimated to have Parkinson's disease.

A higher incidence of Parkinson's disease has been found in persons who live in a rural setting in comparison to those who live in the city. Dr. Jean Hubble showed a higher occurrence of Parkinson's disease in residents of rural western Kansas compared to those who lived in the city, and other similar studies have confirmed this observation.

◈ RISK FACTOR: TOXIC ENVIRONMENTAL EXPOSURES

People who have drunk from well water and who have been exposed to herbicides and pesticides appear to be at greater risk of developing Parkinson's disease. This may explain the higher risk of Parkinson's disease in rural and farm areas, versus those who live in the city. A study on rats that were chronically exposed to rotenone, a chemical found in many pesticides, found that the exposure caused the development of rigidity and slowness and loss of dopamine brain cells similar to that seen in human Parkinson's disease.

Parkinson's disease has also been shown to be more common in industrialized nations and among persons employed in vegetable farming, paper mills, and chemical-, copper-, and iron-related industries. In addition, the amount of iron and aluminum content has been reported to be much higher in the brains of people with Parkinson's disease. Prolonged occupational exposure—exposure lasting twenty years or more—to a combination of heavy metals, including copper, lead, iron, and manganese, has been reported to increase the relative risk of acquiring Parkinson's disease to as much as 10 times that of the normal population.

Exposure to carbon monoxide, carbon disulfides, and other organic solvents is also associated with a greater occurrence of Parkinson's disease. One patient, Bobby, was only 13 years old when he developed classic signs and symptoms of Parkinson's, with tremor, rigidity, and slowed movements. When searching for clues as to why he got Parkinson's disease at such a young age, his physicians discovered that he and his father had been poisoned from carbon monoxide when he was 8 years old. The level of carbon monoxide in their home was too high, and both were taken to the hospital and seemed to have survived without any problems. His father had not shown any signs of Parkinson's disease, nor was there anyone known to have the disease in his family. But it certainly was a possibility that the carbon monoxide was toxic to Bobby's brain cells and triggered the Parkinson's disease that showed up only five years later.

In cases like Bobby's, when a suspected toxic agent is identified, it is almost impossible to prove that prior exposure to such a toxin is the sole cause of Parkinson's disease. No specific test can prove this. Physicians simply rely on the history and look for what's known as a "temporal" link, meaning the onset of Parkinson's disease is linked in time to the time of exposure to the toxin. However, this method does not always work, especially since up to 60 to 70 percent of the dopamine brain cells must stop functioning before the motor symptoms of Parkinson's disease are detected. What that means is that Parkinson's disease may not be readily diagnosed until many years after exposure to an agent, as in the case of Bobby, where five years elapsed between exposure to a toxin and the appearance of symptoms.

❖ RISK FACTOR: VIRAL INFECTIONS

Viral infections have been implicated as a possible cause of Parkinson's disease. As mentioned earlier, the World War I outbreak of sleeping sickness resulted in physical symptoms similar to Parkinson's disease. (The movie *Awakenings*, starring Robin Williams, was based on this story.) However, after examining the brains of some of these patients at autopsy, it was found that this sickness was not true Parkinson's disease, but rather a viral brain infection that had some of the same clinical symptoms.

A few studies have supported the possibility of an infectious cause of Parkinson's disease, showing higher incidence of nocardia infection and corona virus antibody in the cerebrospinal fluid (fluid that covers the brain) in patients with Parkinson's disease. However, unlike other viruses or infectious diseases, Parkinson's disease isn't isolated to a specific geographic region or a specific generation or time period. Also, most infectious diseases are seen to spread via epidemic. Since Parkinson's disease has never acted in a true epidemic fashion, it's hard to support the theory that Parkinson's disease is solely or primarily part of an infectious process.

❖ RISK FACTOR: MPTP

MPTP is a man-made chemical that was directly linked to acute Parkinson's disease in young persons in the 1980s in Northern California. IV drug users who bought and used synthetic heroin that contained MPTP arrived in the emergency rooms with acute and severe muscle rigidity, bradykinesia, and tremors. Some of these patients did not survive, and autopsy reports showed complete loss of the dopamine brain cells in the same area of the brain—the substantia nigra—as seen in typical Parkinson's disease. This chemical has since been used to create animal models for the study of Parkinson's disease in rats and primates. It is not found or readily available except in laboratories, where it is manufactured for research purposes. Studies of MPTP have, however, led scientists to develop the theory that a defect in the mitochondria—the cell's energy producer—may play a part in the development of Parkinson's disease.

❖ RISK FACTOR: ESTROGEN DEFICIENCY

Estrogen may act as a neuroprotective agent in Parkinson's disease. A report in the journal *Movement Disorders* compared the medical records of seventy-two women who were diagnosed with Parkinson's disease to women of the same age who did not have Parkinson's disease. The results showed the women who were diagnosed with Parkinson's disease had

- A significantly higher rate (almost three times) of hysterectomies;
- A higher rate of early menopause; and
- A lower rate of using estrogen replacement hormones after menopause.

These findings, along with the lower rate of Parkinson's disease in women in general, certainly suggest that estrogen or other female hormones may help protect dopamine brain cells and prevent or delay the onset of Parkinson's disease. Clearly, they alone do not prevent it, as many women still get Parkinson's disease, but a clue may be hidden somewhere in the world of female hormones about what causes Parkinson's disease or about future treatments.

◈ RISK FACTOR: GENETICS

Chromosomes are the genetic material or blueprints that we all inherit from our parents. They determine many things about us, including the color of our eyes, our gender, height, and many other physical characteristics, including the potential to develop certain illnesses, such as cancer, diabetes, high cholesterol. Chromosomes are made up of DNA (deoxyribonucleic acid), and within the DNA are genes, the components responsible for the many traits that we inherit.

When deciding whether a disease is inherited or not, an accurate family history is extremely important. This is especially the case with first-degree relatives—parents, siblings, and children. The greater number of people in a family with Parkinson's disease, the more likely it is that a genetic factor exists. It has been estimated by some experts that only 10 to 15 percent of persons with Parkinson's disease report a positive family history of Parkinson's disease in first-degree relatives. This suggests that 85 to 90 percent of persons with Parkinson's disease do not have other family members who are also affected. This and other similar reports have led many to believe that Parkinson's disease is for the most part not an inherited disorder, but rather a sporadic disease of unknown cause. There are, however, other studies that have reported that as many as 35 to 40 percent of Parkinson's patients have first-degree relatives who have the condition.

The debate over whether Parkinson's disease is genetically determined is far from over and is starting to heat up. Some experts believe that because more than two-thirds of the cells in the substantia nigra need to be lost before a person exhibits symptoms of Parkinson's disease, some family members related to a person with Parkinson's disease may actually have the condition themselves but do not show the physical symptoms or signs because they have lost only 30 or 40 percent of the dopamine brain cells. This is called subclinical or preclinical Parkinson's disease. It is possible that these family members may die from some other cause such as heart disease, cancer, or trauma well before they develop symptoms or are diagnosed with Parkinson's disease. The prevalence of undiagnosed subclinical Parkinson's disease may mean, therefore, that the influence of genetic factors is underestimated.

Despite the large number of people with Parkinson's disease who lack a positive family history, there are rare families where multiple family members across several generations have Parkinson's disease. Studies by geneticists analyzing the DNA of the members of these families have identified specific regions on the chromosome or certain genetic variants that cause Parkinson's disease in these patients. Perhaps the most famous family with inherited Parkinson's disease is the Contursi family, described by Dr. Golbe in 1990, in which sixty members of the same family over five generations were diagnosed with Parkinson's disease. Two persons who died had autopsy reports that showed the classic loss of dopamine cells and the presence of Lewy bodies found in Parkinson's disease. Later studies by Dr. Mihael Polymeropoulos in 1996 and 1997 found a particular genetic mutation on chromosome number 4 to be the genetic cause of Parkinson's disease in this family.

Many other chromosome mutations have recently been identified in families with Parkinson's disease, including those on chromosome numbers 1, 2, 4, 6, and 12. It is quite possible that the world of genetics will unravel the mystery as to what causes Parkinson's disease and ultimately pave the way for neuroprotective and curative treatments in the future. The role of genetics in the future of Parkinson's disease diagnosis and treatment is explored further in chapter 11.

What Are the Chances That Your Children Will Get Parkinson's Disease?

While there is no firm statistics on this, the following chart is considered to be a good estimate of the risk.

Risk of Getting Parkinson's Disease Based upon Family History of Parkinson's Disease

Person with Parkinson's Disease in Your Family	Chance of Getting Parkinson's Disease
None	1–2%, same as general population
Brother or Sister	5–6%
Parent only	10%
Parent and Brother or Sister	20–40%

If you do have other family members with Parkinson's disease, your chances of getting Parkinson's disease are greater than the general population, but this does not necessarily mean that you will get Parkinson's disease. And if you currently do have Parkinson's disease, but no one else in your family does, it is more likely your children will not develop the condition in their lives. Even in cases where a parent and a brother or sister have been diagnosed with Parkinson's, it is still more likely that the child of that parent will not get Parkinson's disease.

Greg was only 43 years old when he was diagnosed with Parkinson's disease.

> My father was diagnosed with Parkinson's disease five years ago at age 60, and I have a first cousin with it and one aunt, my father's sister, who also has it. I'm very worried that my children will inherit Parkinson's disease from me. I've decided to participate in a genetic study, as has my family. It involves giving a couple of blood samples so the scientists can look for a gene in my family that might be the cause of Parkinson's disease. I think it's important to try to figure out what causes Parkinson's disease, and if a little bit of my blood can help, then I will gladly give it. I know it won't probably change my diagnosis or treatment, but it might help for future treatments and I feel like I'm making a difference.

Risks for Twins

Recent studies on twins with Parkinson's disease have shown very little risk of the twin getting Parkinson's disease when his or her identical twin had been diagnosed with the condition. However, the relative risk of getting Parkinson's disease in the symptom-free twins increased almost six times if the onset of Parkinson's disease occurred before age 50 in the symptomatic twin. This argues that there may be more of a genetic risk for young-onset Parkinson's as opposed to Parkinson's disease that develops later in life. Alternatively, one could argue that because it takes time to develop symptoms, twins who are younger have a greater likelihood than twins who are older of both twins showing the physical symptoms of Parkinson's disease in their lifetime. This again suggests subclinical Parkinson's disease, where someone has the condition but the symptoms are not yet evident. PET scans of the brain have actually shown loss of dopamine cell function in a symptom-free identical twin of a Parkinson's disease patient. It seems the role of genetics in Parkinson's disease is still being defined, and future studies will allow for an accurate definition to be written.

OTHER FACTORS

Caffeine

Caffeine has recently been reported to be associated with a lower occurrence of Parkinson's disease. In a study published in the *Journal of the American Medical Association*, it was reported that the risk of Parkinson's disease in those who don't drink coffee was five times greater than those who drank 28 ounces—approximately three cups—per day of caffeinated coffee. Similar findings were reported in another study where a later age of onset of Parkinson's disease occurred in persons who drank coffee (72 years) compared to those who did not (64 years).

One must be cautious when reading such reports, however, as it's easy to jump to false conclusions. Does this mean that something in coffee protects brain cells from dying? Probably not, but it does provide researchers something to think about and investigate further to prove whether there is any real meaning behind this observation.

So should you start drinking coffee? At this point, practitioners are not recommending it to prevent or treat Parkinson's disease. Also, be aware that drinking over three to four cups a day may cause unwanted symptoms of worsening tremor, an increased need to urinate, diarrhea, nausea, vomiting, headaches, anxiety, and insomnia.

Nicotine/Cigarettes

It has also been reported that lower rates of Parkinson's disease occur in patients who smoke cigarettes. It has been speculated that nicotine may have a neuroprotective property and protect dopamine cells from dying. In research, nicotine was shown to protect against MPTP-induced dopamine cell death in rats in several studies. However, this is certainly not proof that nicotine prevents Parkinson's disease. It was thought that maybe people who smoked died sooner, perhaps before they developed cigarette-related illnesses—cancer, heart disease—long before the onset of Parkinson's, but studies have shown this not to be the case. Current speculation is that nicotine may regulate the release of dopamine in the brain and may improve memory and thinking. However, a recently reported double-blind study with a nicotine patch in persons with Parkinson's disease showed no improvement in the motor symptoms of those who used the nicotine patch compared to those who received a placebo patch with no active nicotine. Like caffeine, the issue of cigarette smoking and its relationship to Parkinson's disease remains poorly understood. (Note from Dr. Jill: Don't even ask if this means you should start smoking cigarettes or if you currently smoke that you shouldn't stop!)

Diet and Nutrition

Although the results of many studies on diet and Parkinson's disease are controversial and no definite dietary factor has been identified as a cause of Parkinson's disease, there is at least the suggestion and possibility that diet may play a role in the cause of Parkinson's disease or in the treatment and prevention of it.

An abundance of free radicals and other possible toxins such as iron are believed to play a role in dopamine cell death. Hence, diets that promote excess free radicals or other toxins could be risk factors for Parkinson's disease. On the other hand, diets rich in antioxidants—such as the vitamin E, vitamin C, and beta-carotene found in fresh fruits and vegetables—could decrease the presence of free radicals and potentially reduce one's risk of getting Parkinson's disease.

In fact, several controlled studies showed a lower occurrence of Parkinson's disease in patients who had a diet rich in vitamin E, or who took vitamin E, multivitamins, and cod liver oil, or who took vitamin C. However, other similar studies have failed to support this. Other smaller studies have reported a lower occurrence of Parkinson's disease with diets rich in nuts, vegetables, and niacin, and one showed a higher risk of Parkinson's disease with diets rich in animal fat.

Note from Dr. Jill: The Parkinson's Personality

Among practitioners who work regularly with Parkinson's disease, many of us have found that the majority of Parkinson's patients have a similar personality type. While it doesn't apply to everyone, in general, Parkinson's patients tend to be particularly "nice" and to have a diligent, trustworthy, and loyal character and somewhat reserved demeanor. The Parkinson's disease patient is not normally considered to be a risk taker but is reliable—someone you can count on. In fact, I noted this during my neurology residency, and one of the reasons I chose to study Parkinson's disease was my attraction to the patients and their caregivers. Overall, they are a delightful group of people to get to know and to care for. People with Parkinson's listen and follow advice often to the letter, they keep their appointments, they take their medicine, and they come prepared with questions and often know the answers from their own reading and investigation. They tend to be positive, hardworking, and caring people, as do their spouses.

How is it that a personality type might be linked to a particular illness? Is it genetic or biologic? Is it a consequence or reaction of having to cope with a serious illness that changes one's perspective on life? Does this personality in some way predispose one to the development of Parkinson's disease? I don't know, but I do know that my colleagues and I are the benefactors of such personalities and of the many patients we are blessed to know and serve.

Note: A detailed "Risk Factors and Symptoms Checklist" that you can print out and bring to your doctor is available online at www.docjill.com.

Chapter 3

Symptoms and Signs of Parkinson's Disease

Whatever makes us jump back seems at the very least worthy of being examined carefully for its potential usefulness.

—*Clarissa Estes*

While the signs and symptoms of Parkinson's disease can vary greatly among individual patients, Parkinson's disease affects primarily the motor system of the brain and results in difficulty with motor function or movement of the body. These motor symptoms are thought to develop directly due to low dopamine levels, but medicine doesn't have a clear grasp of how these symptoms specifically occur.

There are three primary motor symptoms of Parkinson's disease, and most patients will have at least two of these three key symptoms:

- **Tremor:** a rhythmic oscillation of a body part, such as a hand shaking back and forth with extension and flexion of the wrist

- **Rigidity:** a persistent and relatively constant tightening and stiffening of muscles that can be felt by an examiner and sensed by a patient as muscle stiffness
- **Bradykinesia:** slowness of movement

A fourth symptom—postural instability—is also common in Parkinson's disease. This refers to a decrease in the ability to balance, especially while standing, that often results in patients stumbling or falling. Postural instability is not considered one of the key motor symptoms in diagnosing Parkinson's disease, however, because it is also common in old age and may be related to a variety of other conditions in addition to Parkinson's disease.

The motor symptoms of Parkinson's disease tend to be present on one side of the body more than the other—either left or right. Although most people with Parkinson's disease will eventually develop signs and symptoms on both sides, most patients will have more symptoms on one side versus the other.

In addition to these key motor function symptoms, other parts of the body that may be affected by Parkinson's disease include the skin; eyes and vision; the autonomic nervous system, such as blood pressure, digestive tract, sexual and urinary systems, and body temperature; and cognitive or mental processing.

Keep in mind that if you have some of the symptoms reviewed in this chapter, it does not necessarily mean that you have Parkinson's disease. Several other illnesses, discussed in chapter 4, can cause similar symptoms and be mistaken for Parkinson's disease. However, if you do have many of these symptoms or signs, it's recommended that you be evaluated by a neurologist—or even better, by a Parkinson's disease specialist—to assist with proper diagnosis. And if symptoms persist despite treatment, some additional treatments and suggestions are presented in chapter 9.

◆ EARLY SYMPTOMS OF PARKINSON'S DISEASE

Before a diagnosis of Parkinson's disease is made or is obvious to the patient or physician, patients may experience some of the following early symptoms.

- Fatigue or decrease in energy
- Muscle aches and pains
- Mild slowing or less coordinated performance of simple motor tasks (buttoning, tying shoes, putting on socks/stockings)
- Micrographia (smaller handwriting)
- Constipation
- Depression
- Mild dragging of one leg or a decrease in arm swing while walking
- Seborrheic dermatitis—a red, scaly rash most commonly found on the face or chest

Nathan, a Parkinson's disease patient, describes his early symptoms.

> Looking back, I really think I had symptoms for at least five years before my doctors diagnosed me with Parkinson's disease. My wife and my family doctor thought I was depressed, but I didn't feel depressed, I just felt run down and out of energy. My left foot would cramp in the morning and I felt clumsier when

I tied my tie and when I shaved. Every once in a while my left thumb would quiver just a little and then several years later I began to have more obvious tremors of my thumb. Now that I know what some of the symptoms are, I definitely had Parkinson's disease long before anyone figured it out. My handwriting got tinier and tinier. Eight years later and after a rheumatologist and two neurologists, I was finally diagnosed.

Alice describes the early symptoms her husband, a Parkinson's patient, showed before his diagnosis.

He had been having increasing signs of what we thought at first were small strokes. It began with trouble getting into his wallet with his left hand, not being able to turn the key in the door, etc. We thought maybe carpal tunnel? Maybe mini-strokes? But then the more I watched him, the more I noticed. . . . Some things you just take for granted when you have only known a person for a few years; you think that is just the way they are. But then as I really paid attention I noticed his stuttering getting worse, trembling, his walk became more limpy, then I began to notice when I would call his name, he would turn to me very slack-jawed and seemed to stare right past me at times, like he couldn't comprehend what I was saying.

After several evaluations and an MRI, which ruled out stroke and a brain tumor, he was diagnosed.

❖ MOTOR SYMPTOMS AND SIGNS OF PARKINSON'S DISEASE

Each person will vary considerably in his or her presentation of Parkinson's disease. Some people will have little or no tremor, some will primarily have difficulty with gait and balance, while others will have marked rigidity and slowness. Some patients have a rare form of Parkinson's disease called tremor-predominant Parkinson's disease. With this condition, the person will have very obvious tremors with no rigidity, bradykinesia, balance difficulties, or gait problems.

It is also important to understand that the signs and symptoms of Parkinson's will vary over the course of a day and over the course of one's life. At times, movements may be slower and tremors worse, versus other times, when it may seem as though a person doesn't even have Parkinson's disease. This is due in part to the medications and other therapies that help to lessen these symptoms. When the medicine is working, the person with Parkinson's disease can often feel normal with his or her movements. However, if the medicine has worn off or not had enough time to work, or when a person is tired or emotionally or physically stressed, the Parkinson's disease motor symptoms can worsen. As a Parkinson's patient ages, motor symptoms may also worsen, due to the slow progression of Parkinson's disease.

Riley describes some symptom fluctuations that were treatable by a change in medicine.

I feel pretty good all day; the medicine helps control the tremors and lets me move normally, except in the morning when I wake up. That's the worst time of day for me. I am taking controlled-release Sinemet three times a day. It works great, but I didn't know that it takes two hours before it starts to work until I talked to my neurologist. She told me to add an immediate-release Sinemet to the morning dose of the controlled-release pill, and that did the trick. Now I can move much better in the morning—it only takes thirty minutes to get moving well instead of taking two to three hours.

Tremor

In general, tremor usually begins on one side of the body, and may or may not spread later to the other side. You may notice tremor in the arm, but it can also be seen in the leg and chin or jaw. Rarely, tremor can affect the head or voice.

In very early Parkinson's disease, a mild, intermittent rest tremor—a tremor that occurs only while the person is not using the limb and is relaxed—may occur, typically in the arm, wrist, or fingers. A rest tremor of Parkinson's disease lessens or stops with movement of the affected limb.

Tremor may also occur with a person's arm or leg extended and held up against gravity, and this is known as a postural tremor. Postural tremor is frequently noticed when reading the newspaper or a book or carrying something.

Tremor that occurs when the person uses his or her arm or leg is known as an action tremor, and is rare in Parkinson's patients. Action tremor may be noticed when writing or using a fork or knife to eat or when applying makeup or shaving or doing anything that involves movement of the affected limb.

If an action tremor is present, it usually is not severe or disabling as it might be in essential tremor. Essential tremor is a different condition than Parkinson's disease, and involves tremor primarily with the use or extension of limbs. Essential tremor differs from Parkinson's disease in that it never occurs at rest, and usually involves shaking of the limbs and may involve the head and voice.

A classic Parkinson's disease symptom is a form of tremor known as a "pill-rolling" tremor, which involves a rhythmic rolling movement of the thumb against the index finger, as if rolling a pill between the fingers.

Tremor often worsens with emotional or physical stress and will vary throughout the day, sometimes absent or barely visible, while at other times very evident.

Doctors should always examine for tremor in three ways: at rest; with posture—your arms and legs held out against gravity; and while you use your arms and legs (i.e., the doctor should have you move your finger to your nose, then back to the doctor's finger, then back to your nose).

It is important to note that up to one-third of all Parkinson's disease patients may not have tremor, so lack of tremor does not preclude a diagnosis of Parkinson's disease.

Pat says this about her husband, who was diagnosed with Parkinson's disease:

I noticed my husband's left foot would tremble when he would sit in his La-Z-Boy chair and watch football. When he got up or moved it to stand or walk, it went away.

Merideth says this about tremor:

I have always had tremor. At first it really bothered me. I was so self-conscious and embarrassed. People would stare at me in public. Then they would make me nervous and I would shake even more. The medicines have helped some, but I still shake a good part of the day. Now that I have had Parkinson's for over seven years, I have adjusted and it doesn't bother me as much as it used to or I should say that I don't let the people that stare at me bother me as much.

Rowland shares his humorous view after ten years of dealing with Parkinson's and its resulting tremor.

I have tremor in both my arms and legs and sometimes in my chin. It used to drive me nuts. Whenever you least want it to show up, it does. So one day I am at Wal-Mart shopping and I was a little late in taking my medicine and of course I forgot to bring it with me and I start shaking away. Well, this lady kept looking at me and she finally comes up to me and says, "Can I ask you why you shake so much?" And I say, "Yes, I have Parkinson's disease," and then I notice that her right hand is shaking too. Then she says, "Oh, thank God, I thought it was cancer!" Then we both laughed!

Rigidity

Rigidity may be felt by a person with Parkinson's disease as muscle stiffness, cramps, or aches and pains in the limbs, trunk, or neck. Some people with Parkinson's disease will have little or no rigidity, whereas others may have severe muscle stiffness. A doctor may detect rigidity by moving an arm or leg around a fixed point, such as flexing and extending the forearm about the elbow or slowly rotating the wrist in a circular pattern.

As with tremor, rigidity is typically more pronounced on one side. It may be present in the arms and legs as well as the neck and back muscles. A particular type of rigidity found in Parkinson's disease is "cogwheel" rigidity, which has a ratchet-like quality that results from a combination of tremor and tightening of muscles.

Adam describes the rigidity he felt:

It was a feeling of tightening in my legs and my neck mostly. If it is really bad, it hurts kind of like when you have a charley horse. It is definitely worse if I forget to take my medication. The medicines definitely help, but every once in a while I have to take an extra pill that relaxes the muscles.

Bradykinesia

Most people with Parkinson's disease have some degree of bradykinesia—a slowness of movement—that can appear in a variety of ways. Patients and physicians sometimes misinterpret the signs of bradykinesia as weakness of the affected side. Some medical conditions, such as a stroke, can make muscles weaker. But the part of the brain involved in Parkinson's disease does not involve motor pathways that cause motor weakness. It does, however, cause slowness and stiffness that can be perceived by patients as a feeling of weakness but is not actual weakness. However, the difficulty experienced in using a limb and the time it takes to exert normal effort with muscles can give the false impression that the muscles are weak.

Bradykinesia can present in a variety of ways. The presence of the following symptoms, explained below, are suggestive of bradykinesia:

- Difficulty with fine motor tasks
- Difficulty initiating movement
- A change in gait or walking
- Freeze attacks
- Masked face
- Micrographia
- Hypophonia

DIFFICULTY WITH FINE MOTOR TASKS

People with Parkinson's disease may have difficulty with buttoning, tying shoes, putting on socks or stockings, applying makeup, shaving, or doing other tasks that require fine motor coordination.

Melanie describes her experience:

I sometimes need help to tie my shoes and button my shirt. It is especially difficult to get my right arm into my sleeve. I gave up stockings three years ago. Who needs them when you live in Florida? I've found that waiting a good hour after taking my medicine in the morning makes it easier to get dressed.

Roy, a surgeon, shares his experience:

Luckily, I was going to retire next year. I'm a general surgeon and I've begun to have trouble using my hands to operate. Even though the medicine makes it better, I have decided to retire seven months ahead of schedule.

DIFFICULTY INITIATING MOVEMENT

Many people with Parkinson's disease will have a hard time turning over in bed or getting up out of a bed, rising from a chair, and getting out of a car. Even in the early stages of Parkinson's disease, they may have difficulty or need assistance in these or other activities that involve initiating movement.

Some patients can demonstrate fairly rapid movement with their hands and feet while sitting in a chair, but when they stand up and begin to walk, they appear to be stuck. Their feet literally won't move, even though their brains are telling them to do so. This is called start hesitancy. Often after a few seconds or minutes, which can seem like hours to the patient, he or she can begin to walk.

Amanda tells of her difficulty with getting started:

> I was diagnosed with Parkinson's over twenty years ago. I am still living on my own, and for the most part able to care for myself, except that I am definitely slower. It has gotten a lot harder to get out of bed in the morning, and I live alone. My doctor helped me to get a metal frame, I think they call it a trapeze, that goes over my bed and has a handle that hangs down so I can grab it and pull myself up. That and silk pajamas (to eliminate friction) and leaving my medicine on the nightstand so that I can take it when I wake up, allow me to get up in the morning.

A CHANGE IN GAIT OR WALKING

Most but not all people with Parkinson's disease will experience some degree of difficulty with their walking. This may simply be a slight slowing of the rate of walking or might involve dragging of one leg. Some patients will walk with very tiny steps and tend to shuffle, even to the extent that they slide their shoes across the floor without picking up their feet.

Many people with Parkinson's disease will have a decrease in the swing of their arms when they walk, with one arm swinging or moving less than the other. This can contribute to balance problems.

Associated with start hesitancy, some people with Parkinson's disease have difficulty when they want to start walking because the feet will not move when they want to begin.

An increase in the speed of forward steps and tendency for the body to propel forward, called festination of gait, can occur and cause a person to lose balance and possibly fall forward. The person appears to be almost running, but with small steps and without fully picking up his or her legs. We take our natural walking ability for granted, and to take a normal stride of two to three feet involves a complex series of motor circuits firing and requires a quick and coordinated movement. Festination occurs because it takes more time to take a big stride, and it's almost as if a Parkinson's patient takes a stride and then it's cut short in midstream, and the total distance of one stride to the next is shortened, sometimes to the point that it's almost two to three inches. While the person with Parkinson's disease is trying to walk as if the body can go as quickly as normal, the body may only be able to take steps of a few inches, which then appears as the festination.

Frequently, patients with Parkinson's disease, especially upon standing, will tend to retropulse—move or fall backward—sometimes even falling back into a chair. Or, when walking, some patients propulse, which means they lean far forward over the feet when walking or festinating. These tendencies, known as retropulsion and propulsion, greatly increase the risk of falling.

It is common in Parkinson's disease to develop a stooped posture with shoulders hunched forward. This may be more noticeable while walking and can contribute to balance problems.

Lyvonne shares her difficulty with walking:

> I used to be a long-distance runner. I have had Parkinson's for almost eight years now and the worst part of it for me is that my right leg gets stuck—it's hard to get it to move when I start to walk and then when I finally get going it drags a little. I have given up running except for on a treadmill, where it is safer. The strange thing is that even though it's hard to walk fast or run, I can dance just like before. I am grateful for that because I love to dance.

FREEZE ATTACKS

Some Parkinson's patients notice that sometimes they suddenly freeze or halt without warning in the middle of walking and it may take a few seconds or minutes to get started again. These "freeze attacks" tend to occur more often when attempting to walk through smaller spaces, such as doorways, or when completing a turn. "Turning en bloc" is the term used to describe a person with Parkinson's disease who needs to take several extra steps to complete a full 180-degree turn, such that it appears he or she is turning on a square (hence the term *bloc*) or in a semicircle, rather than rotating in place.

MASKED FACE

A masked face refers to a reduction in facial expression. It may be mild, or it can be more pronounced. One manifestation of this symptom is an unblinking stare, sometimes described as similar to a reptilian stare. This blank stare can often be misinterpreted by family and health care providers as depression or anger.

Gina described this symptom in her husband:

> I noticed my husband, Kent, would just stare, he rarely smiled, and he didn't blink his eyes at all. I thought he was mad or depressed. That was two years before he was diagnosed with Parkinson's disease. I wish I had known then that it was the Parkinson's disease causing his face not to move.

MICROGRAPHIA

Micrographia is small handwriting. As a person with Parkinson's disease continues to write, the height and width of the letters often decrease. This may be very mild or quite severe, such that the letters are so small one can barely read them. To check for micrographia, one should have unlined paper and start writing at the top of the paper and continue to write down the entire page.

Richard describes the micrographia he experienced:

> I am a journalist, of all things, what a cruel joke it was to get Parkinson's. The first thing I noticed was my handwriting was getting smaller and it took me longer to take handwritten notes. Thank goodness for medi-

cine and for computers. My laptop and my Mirapex keep me writing.

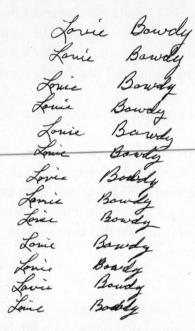

Figure 3. An example of micrographia. The final signature is almost half the size of the first.

HYPOPHONIA

Hypophonia is a reduction in the volume and clarity of one's voice. Hypophonia probably results from a lack of coordination, as well as slowing of vocal cord and respiratory muscles. Some Parkinson's patients may notice that the voice becomes raspier or softer. People speaking on the phone with a Parkinson's patient may complain that the patient's voice is hard to hear.

Steve says that the worst problem from Parkinson's is hypophonia.

> The medicine helps a little, but not enough. It's almost like I'm whispering. When you add this with my wife's hearing problem, it's a wonder that we can communicate at all! But, as she points out, we had that problem way before Parkinson's, like most married couples!

One patient, Harriet, had gotten to a point where she had to write down what she wanted to say in order to communicate. After several months of speech therapy and many years of adjusting her medicine, she got a handheld microphone that allowed her to amplify her voice. This degree of hypophonia is rare, but can occur in some patients.

Postural Instability/Balance Problems

Some people with Parkinson's disease have trouble with balance. Balance problems range from very mild to very severe, with the patient falling on an almost daily basis. The reason behind balance problems is not clear. They may result from rigidity in the muscles of the back that help maintain posture, or they may occur because of the slowed movements, making it harder to quickly correct body position when maneuvering a curve, stairs, or a sudden turn.

Other factors that can contribute to balance problems include a drop in blood pressure, creating a sense of dizziness or light-headedness; dizziness or unsteadiness as a side effect of a host of different medications; poor posture; arthritic joints; tingling or loss of feeling in limbs; and poor vision.

❖ COMMON NONMOTOR SYMPTOMS OF PARKINSON'S DISEASE

Not all people diagnosed with Parkinson's disease will develop the nonmotor symptoms described below. If you do have Parkinson's disease, you may experience none or a few or—rarely—all of these. The key is to be aware that many of these symptoms may have other causes and may not be related to or caused by the Parkinson's disease. A thorough medical evaluation by specialists to rule out other causes and to provide optimal treatment is highly recommended.

Numbness and Pain of the Limbs

Many people with Parkinson's disease complain of numbness and tingling—the medical term for this is paresthesia—as well as pain in their feet and hands. The exact cause of this is unknown, but may be linked to the muscle rigidity thought to be a part of the Parkinson's disease. Other medical conditions—including arthritis and peripheral neuropathy—can cause the same symptoms. Arthritis, however, does not cause muscle stiffness, but rather causes inflammation of the bones and often is detected through blood tests and X-rays of the bones. Peripheral neuropathy is a disorder that results from injury to the nerves that go to the arms and legs and can be diagnosed by nerve conduction studies, which most neurologists can perform.

Skin Changes

Changes in the skin that may be symptomatic of Parkinson's disease include scaling, flaking, and oily skin or seborrhea, a red rash. This is often present in the face and forehead region, especially over the eyebrows and in beards or mustaches. Blepharitis, a rash of the eyelids, can also occur. Some people with Parkinson's disease suffer dry skin that is easily irritated by soaps or clothing.

Vision Changes

People with Parkinson's disease do not have a higher incidence of serious eye diseases, but may experience blurry vision and difficulty focusing. In addition, eye movements may be jerkier, making it difficult to read and to follow moving objects. This may be due to impaired function of the nerves that regulate eye movements and the lens of the eye, as well as due to a loss of dopamine content in the retina, and may also result from side effects of medicine. It is critical for all persons who have Parkinson's disease to get a yearly eye exam to screen for other eye illnesses such as glaucoma and macular degeneration as well as to check visual acuity for proper corrective glasses or contact lenses.

Changes to Sense of Smell

A diminished sense of smell or complete loss of sense of smell is commonly found in people with Parkinson's disease.

Weight Loss

A small percentage of people with Parkinson's disease will have excessive weight loss that is not responsive to dietary changes. This is a symptom that is not well understood. It may be part of a clinical depression, but if adequate trials of antidepressant medications do not correct the weight loss, a more thorough evaluation for other causes should be sought. This would include a complete history and physical to exclude common causes of weight loss such as thyroid disease, cancer, and vitamin and nutritional deficiencies. If weight loss persists and is severe, a nutritional consultation should be sought.

❖ AUTONOMIC NERVOUS SYSTEM (ANS) CHANGES

The autonomic nervous system consists of nerves that regulate the heart rate, contraction and dilation of blood vessels, the digestive tract, sexual organs, body temperature, and virtually all body organs. In some Parkinson's patients, dysregulation of the autonomic nervous system occurs and can result in some or all of the symptoms listed below. These symptoms are rare in the early stages of Parkinson's disease, and may not occur at all at any point in the course of the disease.

Syncope and Presyncope (Fainting and Light-Headedness)

Some Parkinson's patients experience fainting, near fainting, or light-headedness upon standing up. This can occur due to a sudden drop in blood pressure and is known as orthostatic hypotension. Typically, this symptom results from medications that lower blood pressure, including most of the medicines that are used to treat Parkinson's disease. A drop in blood pressure could also indicate a heart condition such as an irregular rhythm; therefore, regular fainting should be evaluated by a cardiologist—and the evaluation should include an electrocardiogram (EKG) and echocardiogram (ultrasound picture of the heart).

Siallorhea (Excessive Saliva)

Siallorhea refers to pooling in the mouth of saliva and drooling. It occurs most likely because of a slowness in the swallowing reflex, which then allows the saliva to build up in the mouth. This may occur to a milder degree during the day, with heavier nighttime drooling, or drooling may be severe and persist throughout the day. This symptom may be very embarrassing socially and can sometimes lead to a skin rash around the mouth known as perioral dermatitis. Less frequently, this excessive saliva can result in breathing in of saliva into the lung and subsequent pneumonia.

Dysphagia (Difficulty Swallowing)

Dysphagia, or difficulty swallowing, can range in terms of severity. It may be mild and occur only with eating large pieces of food, such as meat, or with sticky foods like peanut butter or with especially large pills. Other patients may have more trouble with swallowing thin liquids. If dysphagia is severe, it can result in dangerous choking and may sometimes lead to aspiration pneumonia, where food is lodged in the lung.

Constipation

Constipation, a slowing of bowel movements, is very common in Parkinson's disease and is one of the more common early symptoms. A delay in bowel movements for several days can cause abdominal discomfort and, in severe cases, bowel obstruction. Other factors that can contribute to constipation include medications, a decrease in physical activity, lack of adequate liquid intake, and a low-fiber diet.

Urinary/Bladder Dysfunction

Urinary or bladder dysfunction symptoms include difficulty urinating, an increase in the frequency of needing to urinate, especially at night (known as nocturia), urgency (a feeling of a need to urinate), and less commonly incontinence, a lack of control or unexpected urination without warning.

Breathing

Rarely, people with PD may have difficulty with breathing. This can involve a sense of shortness of breath or shallower breath. A person with PD may breathe as many as 20 to 24 times per minute, when a normal, relaxed breathing rate at rest is 12 to 14 times per minute. This may in part account for hypophonia (decreased volume) in some patients' voices. Patients experiencing breathing difficulties should have a full evaluation by an internist or specialist to rule out underlying heart or lung conditions.

Impotence and Sexual Difficulties

Impotence can be a symptom of Parkinson's disease. Impotence refers to a man's difficulty obtaining and maintaining an erection or, for either sex, difficulty achieving an orgasm. It is also common for both men and women with Parkinson's disease to have a decrease in sex drive, which may be related to low dopamine levels.

Body Temperature Dysregulation

Sudden unexplained hot flashes with flushing or reddening of the skin and excessive uncontrolled sweating, known as diaphoresis, can be a symptom—although it is not common—in people with Parkinson's disease.

◈ MENTAL OR COGNITIVE FUNCTION CHANGES

People with Parkinson's disease may develop difficulty processing information and may have some problems with short-term memory. This is not present early in the course of Parkinson's disease, but may develop during later stages. If the difficulty is severe enough to interfere with daily social and occupational functions, it is called dementia. If the dementia progresses and becomes more severe, the patient may become disoriented to time and place, such that they might get lost walking around the neighborhood or driving familiar roads. They may also not recognize familiar friends or family members and may have difficulty performing simple daily tasks such as dressing, bathing, and cooking.

Dementia has been estimated in 30 percent of all Parkinson's disease patients. Dementia in Parkinson's disease differs from that of Alzheimer's disease (AD) and is usually not as severe. The dementia in Parkinson's disease commonly presents with slowed thinking—known as bradyphrenia—such that it might take the Parkinson's disease person longer to respond, but his or her response may be correct. Parkinson's disease patients with dementia may forget events that occurred earlier in the day, but tend to retain good recollection of events from long ago. Persons with dementia and Parkinson's disease may also have changes in mood or personality, become less animated and motivated, and have a flattened affect, meaning that they express less or little emotion. They may also experience difficulty in processing visual spatial information, such as interpreting a map, and disorientation regarding time and place can occur as well.

As part of a dementia syndrome, people can also have delusions, illusions, or hallucinations. Delusions are fixed false beliefs, such as, "The medicine the doctor is prescribing is actually poison." Illusions are distortion of perception, for example, looking out the window and seeing a tree but thinking it's a person. And hallucinations are perceptions that are not based on reality, typically visual, for example, seeing insects crawling on the wall or children running around the room.

Depression

Depression may occur in as many as 50 percent of people with Parkinson's disease. It typically results from the combination of a reaction to the difficulties of living with Parkinson's disease, along with chemical changes in the brain related to the Parkinson's disease.

People with Parkinson's disease may experience anxiety, intense fear, and panic attacks, often as part of a depression syndrome. Sometimes depression is so severe that people develop delusions and hallucinations. This is called a psychotic depression. The good news is that this is often reversible with the right medications.

Sleep Disturbances

Difficulty with sleep is common among Parkinson's disease patients due to a variety of factors, including a reduction in the amount of time spent in the deep stages of sleep, coexisting depression, urinary frequency at night, and possible side effects from medication, which can sometimes cause nightmares or vivid dreams and, less commonly, hallucinations. In addition to these problems, patients with Parkinson's disease may experience a feeling of inner restlessness called akathisia. The patient feels compelled to move about by walking or marching in place or moving his or her body.

A similar feeling may occur primarily in the legs and is often accompanied by a creeping, crawling, or irritable sensation in the legs, making a person want to get up out of bed and move about, especially at night. This symptom, called restless legs syndrome (RLS), is often relieved by movement but reoccurs when the person lies down again. Another sleep disorder, called REM (rapid eye movement) behavior sleep disorder (RBSD), results in the person physically acting out dreams such that he or she might scream, sit up, punch, kick, or get out of bed. This can sometimes result in injury to the patient or bed partner. People with RBSD are not aware of what they are doing as they are asleep and dreaming.

The primary symptoms of Parkinson's disease are the motor symptoms that may vary considerably from person to person and may fluctuate within one individual over the course of a day and the course of his or her lifetime. Other, nonmotor symptoms may be present to varying degrees as well and, if present and bothersome, should be thoroughly evaluated to look for the cause and to allow for proper treatment.

Note from Dr. Jill

Please don't be discouraged after reading this chapter. The vast majority of patients do not develop all of these symptoms, and most will have only a few. It really is rare for a patient to have a large number of these symptoms. Also keep in mind that effective treatments are available for many of these symptoms.

Chapter 4

Getting a Diagnosis

Health is a state of complete physical, mental and social well-being, and not merely the absence of disease or infirmity.

—*Heave*

Some patients can find that getting a diagnosis of Parkinson's disease is a challenge. Most patients, in fact, have the motor symptoms of Parkinson's disease for up to five years before being properly diagnosed.

There are several reasons for the difficulty in diagnosis. First, there are no diagnostic tests for Parkinson's disease, meaning that a brain scan does not diagnose it. The dopamine cells that die off in Parkinson's disease are in such a small area of the brain that a CT scan, (referred to as a CAT scan), or MRI of the brain is not able to show these microscopic changes, and most patients with Parkinson's disease will have normal brain scans. Also, there is no blood test, brain wave test, or X-ray that can diagnose Parkinson's disease, and the only definitive diagnosis is through postmortem microscopic evaluation of brain cells by a pathologist.

Second, many of the motor symptoms of Parkinson's disease mimic other conditions commonly found in older persons. For example, if a 70-year-old woman with mild arthritis complains of moving slower and having aches and pains and more difficulty getting up out of a chair, it would be reasonable for her family doctor to think these symptoms are due to her arthritis and advanced age. In addition, many patients are misdiagnosed as being depressed. People who are depressed tend to move slower, have less motivation and energy, and can look angry or sad. In Parkinson's disease the facial muscles often slow down, along with other muscles of the body, and the patient is misinterpreted as being depressed. Also, depression can be part of Parkinson's disease, since it often coexists with the condition, making the diagnosis even more difficult and confusing. Other patients may also have been told they had a stroke, when in fact they did not, but rather had Parkinson's disease. The doctors mistook the slowness and stiffness for the weakness that occurs with a stroke.

Third, not all patients with Parkinson's disease have tremor. Although most people associate Parkinson's disease with tremor, up to one-third of Parkinson's disease patients may never develop tremor. This is not well known, and again can lead to misdiagnosis or a delay in diagnosis. One Parkinson's patient repeatedly assured her doctor that she could not have Parkinson's disease because her neighbor had it and he had a tremor, and she never had tremor.

With an absence of definitive tests, the presence of symptoms similar to those found in other conditions, and the confusion over tremor, diagnosis of Parkinson's disease can be complicated. Ultimately, it relies on the physician's performing a detailed history and physical examination, and depends on that physician having a good knowledge base and experience diagnosing Parkinson's disease. Therefore, when Parkinson's is suspected, it is important to seek out neurologists or movement disorders specialists who have advanced training and expertise in diagnosing and treating Parkinson's disease.

◈ DR. JILL: THE STORY OF ROSE

The story of one patient, Rose, illustrates the dangers of misdiagnosis. Rose had had Parkinson's disease symptoms for five years, and they had worsened to the point that she could barely move. In the two weeks before she finally saw me, she had lost the ability to get up out of a chair and could take only a few small steps with someone holding on to her. She began choking on food and she needed help with everything, including dressing, bathing, and eating. Rose had been told that she had had a stroke. Her daughter read a newspaper article that described the signs and symptoms of Parkinson's disease, and she thought to herself, "That's what my mother has." A week later, Rose was in my office. Rose indeed had advanced Parkinson's on examination; she was so stiff that I could barely move her arms and legs, and her daughter and I had to help her to stand up out of the chair. She could not take even one step with us holding on to her, and she had a frozen, expressionless face and a very soft voice. I was so fearful of her falling and choking that I wanted to admit her to the hospital, but Rose wanted to stay home. I agreed to let her go home with twenty-four-hour supervision from her children and arranged for home physical therapy and started her on carbidopa/levodopa.

Before her follow-up appointment in two weeks, the physical therapist called to say she didn't qualify for more physical therapy because she was doing so well. I couldn't believe my eyes when I saw her the next week. She was dressed in a hot pink outfit, had makeup on, and walked into the exam room with ease. Needless to say, we were all delighted. She had very little rigidity, had moderate slowness on the left side and normal facial expression, and could get up out of the chair without help. This was a true awakening of a body and soul. Two years later, Rose is still living independently, has returned to singing in the church choir, and is still a very stylish dresser. "I got my life back, thanks to my daughter and my doctor," says Rose.

❖ THE IMPORTANCE OF EARLY DIAGNOSIS

Rose's story is a good example of why it's critical to have Parkinson-like symptoms evaluated by an experienced neurologist. The earlier you can get a diagnosis, the better, given that some of the drug treatments available may be shown to slow the progression of the disease. Patient advocate Marie Savard, M.D., author of *How to Save Your Own Life* and *The Savard Health Record,* believes that patients should keep a detailed symptoms journal. Says Dr. Savard:

> Often the early symptoms can be missed. Early symptoms can be subtle such as resting tremor, changes in handwriting, difficulty cooking or beating eggs, "frozen shoulder," difficult swallowing, slurred speech or difficulty swinging an arm or an altered gait. A journal will help spot these observations earlier than a doctor would notice. I had a patient who kept a journal of her symptoms, which really helped her neurologist figure out what was going on—things like the description of her tremor, which extremities were involved, medications that she tried, tests that were taken before. . . .

❖ COMMON MISDIAGNOSES

Based on the above, one can understand how it might be difficult to diagnose a person with Parkinson's disease, especially in the early stages. A variety of conditions have similar symptoms to Parkinson's disease and are commonly misdiagnosed.

Arthritis

Arthritis is a condition that affects the bones and joints and typically includes some degree of bone or joint pain. Arthritis can result in obvious enlargement or deformity of joints of the hands, feet, wrists, knees, hips, back, and shoulders. X-rays and certain blood tests are helpful in diagnosing arthritis. As in Parkinson's disease, pain is a common complaint of persons with arthritis. However, while arthritis does cause stiffness of the joints, it does not cause stiffness of the muscles, which is more common in Parkinson's disease. As in Parkinson's disease, balance may be worsened if arthritis involves the knees, feet, or spinal column. In addition, arthritic joints of the hands and knees and low back can cause a person to move slowly and walk slowly and appear to have bradykinesia similar to that seen in Parkinson's patients. Posture may be stooped because of arthritis of the back, again mimicking the stooped posture of Parkinson's disease. Persons who have arthritic hands may have difficulty with fine motor coordination and have micrographia—small handwriting.

The key distinguishing features between arthritis and Parkinson's disease are that in arthritis, resting tremor does not occur and muscle tone is normal. If a patient has some of these symptoms and the doctor suspects arthritis, but X-rays, blood tests, and a physical exam do not readily show arthritis, then the possibility of Parkinson's disease should be considered, and patients should ask for a referral to a neurologist. Another marker is that the aches and pains of Parkinson's disease—typically related to stiffness of the muscles—usually do not respond to the medicines used to treat arthritis. Parkinson's-disease–related pain would usually lessen with use of the medications for Parkinson's.

Depression

Depression may stem from a reaction to something that saddens a person, such as the death of a close friend or family member or any significant adverse event in one's life, such as a career change, loss of a job, breakup of a relationship, etc. Depression that occurs in reaction to an environmental stressor is called exogenous depression. Depression can also occur out of the blue, without warning and without any obvious trigger. This type of depression is called endogenous, meaning that it results from a chemical imbalance in the brain, usually low levels of norepinephrine, dopamine, or serotonin. Endogenous depression is very common, affecting an estimated 20 percent of the general population at any given time. The signs and symptoms of depression are very similar to those of Parkinson's disease and include the following:

- A decrease in facial expression
- Slowed motor movements
- Decreased appetite
- Weight loss
- Lack of motivation
- Slowed thinking
- Difficulty with sleep

- Depressed or angry mood
- Stooped posture with head looking down
- Tearfulness or crying episodes
- Decrease in sexual drive

Since many of these symptoms occur as part of Parkinson's disease, there may be a tendency to diagnose depression, the more common condition, rather than Parkinson's disease. To make matters more confusing, depression often coexists with Parkinson's disease, and may be caused by the depletion of dopamine or other chemicals in the brain.

So, to make an accurate diagnosis, it is very important for the physician to look for objective signs of Parkinson's disease on physical examination. These signs include an obvious tremor, muscle rigidity, and imbalance that would not be caused by depression.

If your doctor has told you that you are depressed, but you don't feel depressed, just slowed down, and you have not improved with adequate medicines that treat depression, then you should be evaluated for Parkinson's disease.

Cindy describes her situation:

I had Parkinson's disease symptoms for at least two years before I was finally sent to a neurologist, who diagnosed it right away. My family doctor and my boyfriend thought I was depressed because I moved so slowly and I would stare. I kept telling everyone that I didn't feel depressed, just out of energy like someone had unplugged me. I tried three different medicines for depression, which helped a little, but they didn't help me move any faster. I wish someone had figured this out sooner so I didn't have to suffer for two years. I was actually glad when the neurologist told me I had Parkinson's, because there was medicine that could help me and because I finally knew what was wrong.

Normal Aging

Normal aging involves a gradual slowing down of movements. Most people who are 70 walk slower than people who are 20. Older people tend to be a little slower in their thinking and may have mild memory problems. They also tend to develop mild changes in posture, and many may have some type of arthritis. Older people often experience a little more difficulty with balance and walking, especially if they have other illnesses such as peripheral neuropathy or arthritis, have impaired vision, or take medicine that can affect their balance or lower their blood pressure. They may also have other serious health problems such as a heart or lung condition that might cause them to move more deliberately. Some older people will develop a mild tremor similar to essential tremor.

So one can see how easy it is to incorrectly assume that a person is suffering from symptoms of aging, attributing the symptoms of Parkinson's disease to "old age." When it's not clear whether a person might have Parkinson's disease or is simply experiencing the effects of being older, and the symptoms of slowness and stiffness and imbalance are disabling, some neurologists will recommend starting a trial course of Parkinson's drugs. If there is no obvious improvement with a good trial of Parkinson's disease medicine (carbidopa/levodopa or a dopamine agonist), then the medicine should be discontinued, with twice-yearly physical exams after that point. If after a year or two of exams no marked worsening of the motor symptoms is observed, then a physician can be fairly confident that the person does not have Parkinson's disease.

Essential Tremor (ET)

Essential tremor (ET) is very different from Parkinson's disease, but because it often involves tremor in the limbs, it is quite frequently confused with Parkinson's disease by physicians, including some neurologists. Essential tremor is actually much more common than Parkinson's disease—almost ten times more common, with over ten million Americans affected by it.

Essential tremor consists only of tremor and lacks the other motor symptoms of Parkinson's disease. There is no rigidity, no bradykinesia, and no balance difficulty in patients with essential tremor. The tremor of essential tremor usually occurs with use of the limbs (action tremor), is bilateral (occurring in both left and right arms or legs), and may occur in the voice (such as in Katharine Hepburn) or the head (such as in Ronald Reagan).

Essential tremor is much more likely to be inherited, with as many as 50 percent of the people with ET passing it on to their children. Many patients will have a parent, and possibly a sibling or grandparent, with a similar tremor. In contrast, it is unlikely that a child of a person with Parkinson's disease will develop the disease as well.

Tremor in essential tremor occurs with the limbs extended—known as postural tremor—and held against gravity and when the limbs are in use. This differs from Parkinson's disease, where tremor is present at rest, when the limbs are relaxed, and typically lessens or stops with use of the limbs. Patients with essential tremor will often complain of difficulty with handwriting, not because it is small as in Parkinson's disease, but because it is difficult to steady the pen and the handwriting is often very sloppy, large, and, in severe cases, illegible. In addition, patients with essential tremor will often spill food off a fork or liquid out of a glass.

It is critical to not be misdiagnosed with essential tremor if you have Parkinson's disease, and vice versa, as both are treatable conditions but are treated with very different medications. Essential tremor typically lessens with alcohol use and responds to beta-blocker medicines as well as mysoline and antianxiety drugs—Parkinson's disease medications usually do not reduce the tremor.

One Parkinson's patient, Scott, was diagnosed with essential tremor for ten years before he saw a different neurologist who diagnosed him with Parkinson's disease.

> The medicine I had been taking for ten years didn't really make a difference in the tremors, but the doctor told me to take it, so I did. I noticed I was getting a little slower with my walking, but thought it was just the changes that happen with an aging 70-year-old body, until I started the Atamet for the Parkinson's. The Atamet made me shake less and I could walk faster without dragging my right leg. I feel like I wasted ten years of being on the wrong medicine. I wish I had seen a specialist back then.

Scott's story is all too common—as is the reverse, when essential tremor patients are diagnosed with Parkinson's disease. It is important for physicians and patients to be aware of the differences between these illnesses in order to ensure proper treatment.

Stroke

Rarely, some Parkinson's patients are misdiagnosed initially as having had a stroke. This usually occurs when a person lacks visible tremor, which is the usual marker physicians look for in Parkinson's disease, and has had a gradual slowing of movement and worsening rigidity that eventually causes difficulty using one side of the body. Typically, a new doctor who does not know the patient does an initial examination, notices that the right or left side of the body is stiff and so slow that it appears to be weak, and makes the diagnosis of stroke.

The typical signs and symptoms of a stroke can vary, but may involve weakness and stiffness on one side of the body. If a person with Parkinson's disease has severe rigidity and bradykinesia, which is usually worse on one side, the patient and the physician might perceive these symptoms as representing a stroke. Stiffness and slowness, when severe, makes it so difficult for the person to move that it looks like weakness, when in fact muscle strength is normal. Also, with a stroke that causes weakness, the reflexes on the affected side are increased, a symptom not typically seen in Parkinson's disease. Stroke symptoms almost always develop quickly over several minutes or hours, which is much different from Parkinson's, where symptoms develop gradually over many years. The brain scan in Parkinson's disease is normal in appearance, whereas the brain scan in a person who has had a stroke is abnormal and should—two days after the onset of stroke symptoms—show a dark spot on a CAT scan or a bright spot on an MRI scan where the stroke occurred. In addition, if a stroke has occurred, then the motor symptoms should not improve with medication for Parkinson's disease.

One patient, Sandy, was misdiagnosed for several years.

I felt weak and clumsy with my right arm and leg, and my balance was off: I had to drag my right leg when I walked and I had a little bit of tremors of my right wrist. I thought I had a stroke, so I called 911 and went to the emergency room. The doctors told me the brain scan was normal and that I looked like I had Parkinson's, so they started me on medicine for it and I went to a rehab hospital to learn to walk and use my right hand better. I stayed on the medicine, Sinemet, and went to see my neurologist every six months. After one year I was a little better and didn't drag my leg as much, and four years later I was no worse and on the same dose of Sinemet that I had started on. That was when my doctor said we should taper off the Sinemet and do an MRI of the brain. I couldn't notice any difference without the medicine, and neither could my doctor, and the MRI showed a small stroke in the left side of my brain.

In Sandy's case, she did have a small stroke that caused her to look like she had Parkinson's disease. The things that supported a diagnosis of stroke were, first, the sudden onset of symptoms and, second, the slight improvement in her motor symptoms over time.

People who have been told they had a stroke, but whose symptoms have gradually worsened over months or years, and particularly those who also have some tremor, should ask for an evaluation by a Parkinson's disease specialist and ask to get an MRI brain scan.

Normal-Pressure Hydrocephalus

Normal-pressure hydrocephalus is a rare disorder that sometimes can present with parkinsonian features but usually is readily distinguished from Parkinson's disease. Normal-pressure hydrocephalus presents with unsteady gait, a change in cognitive functioning (decreased memory or slowed thinking), and urinary incontinence (inability to control bladder function). A brain scan will show an increase in the fluid of the brain—known as hydrocephalus—which is thought to be the cause of the clinical symptoms, while a brain scan of a Parkinson's patient will appear normal. This condition is treatable if caught early on by a neurosurgeon, who typically places a small tube into the fluid system to drain it and relieve the pressure on the brain.

◆ CONDITIONS THAT MIMIC PARKINSON'S DISEASE

In addition to the common misdiagnoses listed above, several other illnesses can be confused with Parkinson's disease. We can lump these conditions into two groups: secondary parkinsonism (when a known cause can be found) and the Parkinson-plus syndromes.

Secondary Parkinson's

Secondary Parkinson's can be caused by medications that block dopamine activity in the brain. The most common of these types of medications are the antipsychotic medicines often used to treat schizophrenia or mania (i.e., haloperidol, chlorpromazine hydrochloride). Antiemetics—the drugs used to prevent nausea and vomiting—such as metoclopramide (Reglan), prochlorperazine (Thorazine), and promethazine hydrochloride (Compazine), and dopamine-depleting drugs such as reserpine and tetrabenazine, can also cause drug-induced parkinsonism. Some of the newer atypical antipsychotics (i.e., clonazepine, quetiapine) are less likely to induce parkinsonism. Stroke and rarely brain tumors involving the area of the brain affected by Parkinson's disease (basal ganglia) and head trauma (as in the case of Muhammad Ali) can also result in secondary parkinsonism.

One patient, Dean, was a 63-year-old CEO of a Fortune 500 company when he was first evaluated for Parkinson's. He had noted a mild tremor of his thumb and some difficulty with writing for six months. During the history taking, he told his doctor he was taking a drug called Reglan for his heartburn. He had been taking this medicine for about six months. His physical exam was consistent with mild Parkinson's disease, but it was possible that the Reglan was causing the parkinsonism. The only way to know would be to stop the medicine and see if his symptoms went away. He stopped the drug, and three months later he was back to normal, without tremors, rigidity, or micrographia (small handwriting). Dean had drug-induced parkinsonism from the Reglan.

Secondary parkinsonian symptoms caused by medication typically improve and reverse within months and almost always by six months. In rare cases, it may take a full year before the person is completely back to normal.

Parkinson-Plus Syndromes

Parkinson-plus syndromes consist of a group of neurodegenerative illnesses that are pathologically and clinically distinct from Parkinson's disease. These illnesses are rare and are some-times difficult to diagnose unless the physician has specialty training in movement disorders. They include progressive supranuclear palsy, striatonigral degeneration, multiple sys-tems atrophy (cerebellar and parkinsonian types), Shy-Drager syndrome, corticobasal ganglionic degeneration, and diffuse Lewy body disease. These syndromes are called atypical Parkinson's because they differ from Parkinson's disease in a number of the significant ways:

- The motor symptoms are very symmetric, with equal in-volvement of the left and right side of the body.
- Tremor is often not present.
- The motor symptoms and disease progress at a more rapid rate, often with marked disability occurring within five years from the onset of the symptoms.
- The motor symptoms do not respond well to the standard medications for Parkinson's disease.
- Balance may be severely affected early on, resulting in fre-quent falling.
- Difficulty with eye movements, speech, and swallowing is common.

Other parts of the nervous system may be affected, such as the autonomic nervous system (ANS), the pyramidal tracts (re-sulting in weakness, spasticity, and increased reflexes) and the cerebellar system (balance center), which is rare in Parkinson's disease.

◆ MAKING A CLINICAL DIAGNOSIS OF PARKINSON'S DISEASE

Given all of the conditions that have similar symptoms, how does a physician make a diagnosis of Parkinson's disease? Diagnosis is made first by understanding the signs and symptoms of Parkinson's disease and then by performing a detailed history and physical examination. In order to make a clinical diagnosis of Parkinson's disease, however, a patient should have at least two out of these three symptoms: tremor, rigidity, and bradykinesia.

If the patient is not started on medication for Parkinson's disease, he or she should be followed closely with frequent physical examinations. In true Parkinson's disease, the signs and symptoms should slowly worsen and become more evident over several years.

Once medication is started, it is very important to note if the motor symptoms benefit from the medication, meaning that a patient's tremor, slowness, and stiffness should improve with proper doses of dopamine-stimulating medications. If the motor function is not improved, either the doses of the medication are too low, or the patient may not have Parkinson's disease, but rather something else that mimics Parkinson's disease.

Patients who find they aren't improving on medication should request a referral to a specialist in Parkinson's disease, if they are not already seeing one.

To summarize, the key criteria a physician looks for in diagnosing Parkinson's disease include

- Two of the three key motor symptoms (tremor, rigidity, and bradykinesia);

- Unilateral onset of symptoms;
- Persistent asymmetry of motor symptoms (one side remains more affected than the other);
- Progression of symptoms and signs over time;
- Very good response to levodopa or dopamine agonist that persists (lasts longer than five years);
- Dyskinesia from levodopa or dopamine agonist; and
- Clinical course over ten years.

PET and SPECT Scanning and Their Role in the Diagnosis of Parkinson's Disease

Positron emission tomography (PET) is a special test that measures blood flow to the brain and can measure the glucose, oxygen, and levodopa or dopamine activity. By radioactively labeling dopa (F-dopa) and injecting it into the vein of a person, the amount of F-dopa that is converted to dopamine in the brain can be measured by the amount of radioactive activity seen on the PET scan. In persons with suspected preclinical Parkinson's disease or those with a questionable diagnosis of Parkinson's disease, this test can be very useful. Persons who have clinical signs of Parkinson's disease have about a 50 percent reduction in F-dopa activity in the brain, compared to persons who do not have Parkinson's disease.

In one study, seven families that each included at least two persons who had been diagnosed with Parkinson's disease were examined, and thirty-two asymptomatic people who had no signs of Parkinson's who were related to the family member with Parkinson's disease had F-dopa PET scans. Almost 30 percent of the family members had a marked reduction of F-dopa activity in the brain, suggesting that they had subclinical Parkinson's disease and were at much higher risk of developing the signs and symptoms of Parkinson's disease in the future. Three years later, three of the eleven persons with abnormal PET scans did develop motor symptoms of Parkinson's disease.

PET scanning is a very expensive test that is not readily available at most medical centers and is therefore not used as a standard diagnostic tool for Parkinson's disease. It is currently used primarily as a research tool. If, however, a drug that delays or arrests the progression of Parkinson's disease becomes available in the future, the importance of diagnosing Parkinson's disease before clinical symptoms appear will become critical and PET scans may play a key role in early or preclinical diagnosis of Parkinson's disease.

SPECT (single photon emission computed tomography) is not as sensitive as PET, but is more widely available and can also measure dopamine activity in the brain in a similar way.

In the course of a second opinion to decide whether to proceed with deep brain stimulation surgery, one patient, Martha, gave her doctor a videotape showing some of her difficult times when she had dyskinesia. After an examination and a review of the video, her physician found that it was not clear whether she had Parkinson's disease. She did not have any rigidity, had normal muscle tone, and exhibited more of a postural, kinetic tremor. Her mother had signs of essential tremor but not Parkinson's. Martha was on very high doses of carbidopa/levodopa (over 2,000 milligrams a day) that could be causing some of her symptoms. After a PET scan was positive for Parkinson's disease, showing a marked decrease in F-dopa activity, it was clear that she did have Parkinson's disease.

◈ WHEN YOU'RE FIRST DIAGNOSED

When you get to a point where you are diagnosed with Parkinson's disease, there are some important things to remember.

Find a Doctor You Can Trust

The most important thing when receiving any diagnosis is to feel comfortable with your doctor. You must feel you can trust your doctor and that your doctor cares about you and will be your advocate. If you do not feel this way, then find someone else—trust your instincts. If you question the diagnosis for whatever reason, get a second opinion and ask your doctor if he or she can refer you to someone who is an expert in Parkinson's disease. If your doctor refuses or seems insulted, find another physician. A doctor should not be threatened by your desire to seek another opinion, but rather should respect this and offer you some assistance in doing so. The physician is there to serve, protect, and help you.

Educate Yourself

It is very important to be informed and to educate yourself about Parkinson's disease. Be a self-advocate. If your doctor does not provide you with written material, request it, and if it is not given to you, find it. Get books, surf the Internet, go to a library, get on the mailing list for a newsletter, go to a support group. The resources appendix to this book has many recommended resources.

Ask Questions

Do not be afraid to ask questions. Write them down as they come to you, and bring them to your next appointment.

Share Your Diagnosis

Share your diagnosis with someone you trust: a friend, a spouse, a coworker, a minister. Do not isolate yourself and deny the diagnosis. Do not be afraid to share your feelings, whether they be anger, denial, sadness, or relief that someone finally told you what was wrong after all this time.

Express Your Feelings

If you feel upset or depressed about the diagnosis, express this to your doctors and your friends and family and consider individual counseling.

> **Note from Dr. Jill: Should I Go to a Support Group?**
>
> Sometimes it is good to avoid going to a Parkinson's disease support group soon after receiving a diagnosis of Parkinson's disease, because of all the anxiety and fear about what this means to you. I often discourage patients just diagnosed from doing so, especially if they are young and have mild symptoms. My concern is that they will see one or two people who are much older and have had Parkinson's disease for over twenty years and are using a walker or a wheelchair and then say to themselves, "Is that what I have to look forward to?" If that is how you would respond, then

don't go. Support groups vary widely: Some include many young working people, while others are predominantly older persons. Some groups focus on talking about their Parkinson's disease, others emphasize education and optimism, and some even serve primarily as a social club. If you want to participate in support, find a group that suits your own style.

❖ THE EMOTIONAL STAGES AFTER RECEIVING A DIAGNOSIS

When first diagnosed with a serious illness, many people will go through several waves of emotions—from pure shock and disbelief to anger and deep sadness. It is important to allow yourself to feel these emotions; they are part of you and you should express them. Be aware that they will come and go and pop up sometimes when you least expect them.

While Parkinson's disease is certainly *not* a terminal illness, Parkinson's patients often go through a grieving process after receiving their diagnosis. Dr. Elisabeth Kubler-Ross outlined five stages of death and dying, which are very similar to the stages many people go through after being diagnosed with an incurable chronic disease such as Parkinson's disease.

Stage I—Denial and Isolation
Stage II—Anger
Stage III—Bargaining
Stage IV—Depression
Stage V—Acceptance
Stage VI—Hope

While Dr. Kubler-Ross stops with Stage V, Acceptance, with chronic disease, it's possible to move beyond that stage to a sixth stage, Hope. It's important to strive for this point, but remember that you cannot get there if you are stuck in the earlier stages. That means it is important to work through whatever stage you are in, and not let yourself get mired in anger or depression, in particular.

❖ PATIENTS WORKING THROUGH THE STAGES

Naomi was 68 and just widowed when she was first diagnosed with Parkinson's disease.

> I was so angry with God at first. I thought, "Isn't it bad enough you took my husband away?" Living alone when you are older is hard enough. Now I have to worry about whether I can take care of myself. In the beginning I used to wish I would just die. I used to pray to God to just take me away in my sleep to be with my husband. I didn't have the strength or will to go on. I felt that way for almost two years after I was diagnosed with Parkinson's disease. I lost thirty pounds and couldn't sleep at night, and I stopped going out with my friends. When I didn't show up to church for the first Sunday in fifteen years, my best friend, Melanie, called on me and took me to my doctor. He put me on medicine for depression and she found a support group and took me to it. I met the nicest people in the world. They gave me hope and I learned a lot about Parkinson's disease and I've learned that it isn't the end of the world. It's now five years since I was di-

agnosed with Parkinson's disease, and I have come a long way.

Stew talks about being angry and in denial and how it almost caused him harm:

> I was so annoyed and mad about having Parkinson's disease at age 45 that I just stopped my medicine one day. I thought, "I don't have this and I don't need this medicine!" I became very confused and disoriented and became slower and stiffer and got all sweaty for a few days. I started my medicine and then felt better. I told my doctor two months later and got a little lecture about not stopping medicine abruptly. In retrospect, it was a dumb thing to do. I really understand other young people who have Parkinson's disease being angry—it just doesn't seem fair to age before your time. I have a degree in psychology, so I understand all the stages of grief, but I am not to acceptance yet. I still have some anger.

Stephanie thinks denial can sometimes be an effective strategy:

> I know I have Parkinson's disease, but I trust my doctor and I am smart, so I won't do anything stupid, but I told my doctor that I have decided that I don't have Parkinson's disease, meaning that I am just going to keep on trucking as though I don't and be positive, so part of me refuses to accept it, and I think that's okay. I think my belief will make me healthier, and I don't really care what other people say.

Danny shares an emotional journey that took him years to come to grips with having Parkinson's disease:

> I was definitely in denial. I wouldn't go to the doctor until I had to get my medicine. I used to hold my left hand when it would shake and tense my muscles to stop the tremors. I was mad at the tremor, mad that it tried to give away that something was wrong with me. After about five years, I started to learn more about Parkinson's disease and met a younger guy who had it too. He helped me because he understood what I was going through. We met online and then met in person. I finally realized one day, just like a lightbulb going off in my head, that I wasn't Parkinson's disease, it was just something that affected my body and that I needed to stop obsessing about it and worrying about it all the time. That's when everything changed—I felt like I was in this fog and then suddenly life was good again.

◆ BEGINNING TREATMENT FOR PARKINSON'S DISEASE

Whether and when to begin treatment with medications is an important decision that should be made by both patient and physician, together. If you have Parkinson's disease and your symptoms are causing difficulty with your daily motor function, so much so that life is difficult and you are losing your independence, then you probably would benefit from a dopamine-stimulating medication. This decision will of course vary with each individual. For example, a 42-year-old nurse who is having difficulty writing in her charts and starting intravenous lines on her patients may need medication to maintain her career, whereas an 80-year-old retired accountant who has a mild tremor in his right arm may not want or need to start medication.

There is a common misconception that delaying medication is important and that you should "save it for later" because it will not work for more than five years. This is simply not true. What is true is that as the disease slowly progresses over time, the motor symptoms worsen over time, requiring an adjustment in the dose, frequency, and number of medications in order to lessen the motor symptoms of Parkinson's disease.

Even if you have decided to hold off on prescription medication, it's important to investigate other therapies, as well as your own health practices and behavior. Do you exercise and eat a healthy diet? Are you getting enough rest, relaxation time, and sleep? Do you have any other health concerns, such as high blood pressure, heart disease, or diabetes, that you need to treat more effectively? Are you under any emotional stress? Are you smoking or drinking too much alcohol? By adopting and maximizing healthy behaviors and minimizing unhealthy behaviors, you can improve your physical and emotional health, minimize your disease state, and achieve optimal wellness.

Alternative therapies, also called holistic or complementary therapies, as well as mind-body approaches, are discussed extensively in chapters 7 and 8 and the epilogue. You can consider using some of these therapies early on in the course of your Parkinson's disease, in place of medication or in addition to medication, as a complement to your treatment.

Jean is 51 years old and worked full-time managing a surf shop at the beach. When she was first diagnosed with Parkinson's disease three years ago, she chose not to start medications. Instead, she decided to take herbal therapies under the guidance of an herbalist, increased the frequency of her exercise to one hour of daily yoga, improved her diet, and began to take antioxidants, including vitamins C and E and beta-carotene. She was able to function until a year ago, when her motor symptoms worsened, making it more difficult to write. She also found herself dragging her left leg and stumbling at times. She started on a low dose of a dopamine agonist, and had a definite improvement in her motor function with the medication. Jean continues her herbal, antioxidant, and yoga therapies. She is a perfect example of combining traditional and nontraditional therapies to achieve optimal wellness and minimize the symptoms of Parkinson's disease.

Part II

CONVENTIONAL
TREATMENTS

Chapter 5

Drug Treatments for
Parkinson's Disease

*Every thing on earth has a purpose, every disease an herb to cure
it, and every person a mission.*
—Morning Dove of the Salish Tribe

Once your doctor diagnoses Parkinson's disease and your
symptoms become disabling enough to warrant medication,
you and your physician will need to decide which medications
are best to treat you.

What was once a relatively simple task is now more complex. Back in the 1940s and 1950s, the only available medications for Parkinson's disease were amantadine (brand name
Symmetrel) and the anticholinergic drugs. But the 1967 discovery of levodopa was a major breakthrough, and that drug is
still considered to be the most potent medication for treatment
of the motor symptoms of Parkinson's disease. Since that time,
eight new medications have been shown to help treat Parkinson's disease, and have been approved for use.

There are general guidelines as to what medications are
best for initial treatment and how best to adjust the dose. But
ultimately, the decision is best made individually by the physi-

cian and the patient. Remember, however, that while Parkinson's medications can help you—for example, improve your motor symptoms—most of the drugs can also cause negative side effects. If a medication is making you feel sick in any way, call the doctor who prescribed it and discuss your options. In addition, if a medication is not making you sick, but it hasn't helped you, then you should also investigate with your physician whether or not you should continue taking it. But never stop taking medications without discussing it with your physician, because some Parkinson's disease drugs have to be slowly tapered off rather than abruptly stopped, to avoid side effects and worsening symptoms.

◈ AN OVERVIEW OF PARKINSON'S DISEASE MEDICATIONS

The medications used to treat Parkinson's disease act to replace, stimulate, or enhance dopamine activity in order to improve motor function. In order for these oral medications to work, they must first be absorbed by the gastrointestinal system (intestines) and then cross the blood-brain barrier, where they can act on the dopamine brain cells. Since pure dopamine does not cross the blood-brain barrier, it must be delivered in the form of levodopa, which can cross into the brain.

The combination of carbidopa and levodopa (Sinemet)—from this point forward, we'll be featuring a drug's generic name first, followed by the brand name in parentheses—is the most potent medication for the treatment of Parkinson's disease. Whereas in the past, levodopa was used alone, today it's known that carbidopa helps prevent the breakdown of levodopa so that it can effectively cross into the brain.

It's important to mention here that many physicians and

patients use the brand name *Sinemet* as a generic term, to refer to any carbidopa/levodopa drug. But there are many different forms and names for carbidopa/levodopa that can be prescribed, including Atamet and Sinemet ER, and they are considered relatively equivalent to Sinemet.

Another class of drugs, known as dopamine agonists—including bromocriptine (Parlodel), pergolide (Permax), pramipexole (Mirapex), and ropinerole (Requip)—have a similar chemical structure to dopamine and can cross the blood-brain barrier and directly stimulate the dopamine receptors.

Other drugs, such as MAOB (monoamine oxidase B) inhibitors and COMT (catecholamine-o-methytransferase) inhibitors like tolcapone (Tasmar) and entacapone (Comtan), help the carbidopa/levodopa function better by preventing the breakdown of levodopa, allowing more levodopa to cross the blood-brain barrier and act on dopamine neurons.

A balance between another chemical in the brain, acetylcholine, and dopamine is upset in Parkinson's disease. Anticholinergic medications—such as trihexyphenidyl (Artane) and benztropine mesylate (Cogentin)—are sometimes used in an effort to restore this balance, and help reduce tremor and rigidity in Parkinson's patients.

◆ DOPAMINE AGONISTS AND CARBIDOPA/LEVODOPA

Carbidopa/levodopa (Sinemet, Atamet) and the dopamine agonists—bromocriptine (Parlodel), pergolide (Permax), pramipexole (Mirapex), and ropinerole (Requip)—are the most effective medications for the treatment of Parkinson's disease. Carbidopa/levodopa is considered the most effective medicine to control tremor, rigidity, and bradykinesia.

One patient, Karen, found that pergolide was the optimal treatment for her Parkinson's disease and allowed her to continue on the job.

I'm taking Permax 0.5 milligrams three times a day. It has almost completely stopped the tremor in my right hand and improved my fine motor coordination. The medicine works so well that I can still work as a computer operator.

Other patients have described the complete elimination of troublesome symptoms once on carbidopa/levodopa. One patient, Luke, described his experience:

Sinemet is the best thing that ever happened to me. Since I have been taking it, I don't even feel like I have Parkinson's disease. I can do all the things I used to do. My handwriting is back to normal and I don't drag my left foot anymore.

One caregiver found that carbidopa/levodopa helped her husband regain a great deal of self-sufficiency.

He is walking so much better since he started taking Sinemet. I don't have to help him get up or to take a shower, and he can dress himself again. Life is so much easier.

Long-term use of carbidopa/levodopa—for example, over five to ten years—is, however, associated with the development of motor complications in as many as 50 to 80 percent of Parkinson's disease patients. The most disabling of these motor complications are the dyskinesias, writhing irregular movements of the arms and legs and sometimes the face, neck, and trunk. At times the dyskinesias are severe and can be more disabling than the Parkinson's disease symptoms themselves.

Because of the side effect of dyskinesia with continued carbidopa/levodopa usage, some physicians try the dopamine agonist drugs first, to delay the start of the use of carbidopa/levodopa. These drugs can be effective in some people. In one study, ropinerole (Requip) was shown to be as effective as levodopa in early stage Parkinson's disease. Another study found Requip more effective than bromocriptine (Parlodel). In one study, which was reported on in 2000 in the *New England Journal of Medicine*, 268 Parkinson's patients were studied. Of that group, 179 were randomly selected to take ropinerole, and 89 received levodopa. After five years, among those patients taking ropinerole, only 20 percent developed dyskinesia, compared with 45 percent of those taking levodopa. Also, among those taking ropinerole who developed dyskinesia, only 8 percent had a severe form, versus 23 percent of those taking levodopa who developed dyskinesia.

In another study, researchers from the Parkinson Study Group (PSG), a joint U.S. and Canadian organization, found that during the first two years, only 28 percent of patients who took pramipexole (Mirapex) developed motor complications, compared with 51 percent of patients who took levodopa. Starting treatment with pramipexole also appeared to delay the onset of motor complications. After two years, 72 percent of patients treated with pramipexole were completely free from motor complications. Dyskinesias developed in 31 percent of the levodopa patients but only 10 percent of the pramipexole patients.

Wearing Off, On-Off

Because carbidopa/levodopa has a shorter half-life than the dopamine agonists—*half-life* refers to the time it takes for the drug to be broken down in the body—patients may experience what's known as "wearing off." Wearing off means that the medication's effects may not last long enough, and symptoms return too quickly. For instance, a patient may have had good control of tremor and slower movements by taking Sinemet 25/100 (25 milligrams of carbidopa and 100 milligrams of levodopa) at 7 A.M., 12 P.M., and 5 P.M. the first five years of having Parkinson's disease, but now may have increasing tremor and slowness at 10 A.M. and 3 P.M., two hours before the next dose of medicine is due. Now the patient needs to take the Sinemet every three hours, at 7 and 10 A.M. and 1, 4, and 7 P.M., to control symptoms.

With these drugs, some patients will have "on-off" phenomena, where one minute the medicine seems to be working and literally the next minute it doesn't. Occasionally there will also be dose failures, times when the medicine just doesn't seem to work at all. These motor fluctuations do not occur in everyone, and overall, carbidopa/levodopa and the dopamine agonists work very well to improve and restore motor function.

Starting with Carbidopa/Levodopa versus a Dopamine Agonist

In several recent studies, dyskinesias occurred less often in patients treated with a dopamine agonist alone (5 percent) compared to levodopa alone (36 percent). In addition, patients treated with a dopamine agonist had less "off times," periods when Parkinson's motor symptoms become disabling, compared to those treated with carbidopa/levodopa. The motor symptoms of tremor, rigidity, and bradykinesia were well controlled with dopamine agonists for up to five years in 30 percent of the patients, to such an extent that they did not need to add carbidopa/levodopa to their medication regimen. These recent findings support the use of dopamine agonists in newly diagnosed patients and in early mild-to-moderate Parkinson's disease, then adding carbidopa/levodopa therapy when the patient's motor symptoms are not adequately controlled by dopamine agonists alone, or when intolerable side effects develop.

Despite the trend to use dopamine agonists as a first-line therapy to lessen the risk of developing dyskinesia, most people with Parkinson's disease will need to add carbidopa/levodopa after three to five years to adequately control the motor symptoms. And a recent study comparing the dopamine agonist, bromocriptine, to carbidopa/levodopa as the first medication used in treatment of 782 persons with newly diagnosed, untreated Parkinson's disease over ten years showed only a slightly lower incidence of moderate to severe dyskinesia in the bromocriptine group. More importantly, the bromocriptine group had worsening motor function compared to the carbidopa/levodopa group, arguing that carbidopa/levodopa can be considered as a first-line therapy over dopamine agonists.

In some cases, when side effects appear from carbidopa/levodopa therapy, the dose can be dropped down, and a dopamine agonist added, in order to alleviate symptoms. One patient, José, was taking Sinemet CR 50/200 three times a day for two years with good control of his key symptoms—a tremor and slowness—but then his head started to bob up and down and sideways about two hours after he took his pill. Says José:

My neurologist explained it was probably because of the Sinemet, so we lowered the dose of the Sinemet to 25/100 three times a day, but then I was too slow and the tremors got much worse, so then we added Mirapex and gradually increased the dose to 1.0 milligram three times a day over two months, and now I'm doing better, no head bobbing and good control of tremor and slowness.

The example of José is very common, in that most patients with PD will have to have frequent adjustments of the medications over the course of their lives. When adjusting the dose of carbidopa/levodopa or the dopamine agonists, it often takes several weeks to several months, as the change in medication needs to be done gradually to avoid side effects. A good rule of thumb is to allow two to four weeks to judge whether the medication change has helped.

Remember too that when making any change in a medication, especially when lowering the dose, there may be temporary worsening of the Parkinson's disease motor symptoms until the patient adjusts to the revised dosage.

Patient Age and Choice of Medicine

Does how old you are make a difference in the medication you should take? In some cases, yes. Parkinson's patients over 70 may be less tolerant of the dopamine agonist medications, due to side effects such as confusion, hallucinations, low blood pressure, nausea, vomiting, and daytime sleepiness. Similar side effects can occur with carbidopa/levodopa, but they tend to be less frequent than with the dopamine agonists. Of the available forms of carbidopa/levodopa—immediate release, controlled release (CR) and extended release (ER)—and the dopamine agonists, no one drug has been proven to be superior to the other. Some doctors prefer one medicine to another, and some patients may respond better to one medicine than another, so to some extent, it is a trial-and-error process. There's no simple way to predict what medicine will work best or cause the least side effects. But one important rule to keep in mind is that your doctor should typically make only one medication change at a time. That way, you can accurately assess whether or not a change in medicine, dosage, or timing has hurt or helped.

Sleepiness is one side effect that seems particularly troublesome to patients. John, for example, was a 78-year-old patient who had had Parkinson's disease for six years and was taking medicine to help with his walking and freezing problems.

> Requip made my drowsy; Mirapex made me even more drowsy . . . I would fall asleep at the kitchen table right in the middle of a sentence, and once I woke up with my face in the cereal bowl. When I took the lowest dose of Permax (0.05 milligrams) only one time, I passed out without any warning . . . bang flat on my face on the family room floor.

John and his physician finally settled on carbidopa/levodopa alone, which he was best able to handle without disabling sleepiness.

Another patient, Earlene, had had Parkinson's disease for about 12 years. Her medicines had been adjusted over five years to the point where she was on three different medications, Sinemet CR, immediate-release Sinemet, Permax, and

Eldepryl. She had wearing off and she had a rare form of respiratory dyskinesia in which she would breathe erratically, with rapid multiple inhalations followed by one long exhalation. Amantadine was added to help with that symptom. Two days after starting the amantadine, her husband, Ralph, called in a panic to say Earlene was holding the shotgun and pointing it at the imaginary burglars (she was actively hallucinating). Luckily, Ralph was able to get the gun and call 911 to have Earlene brought to the hospital, where her hallucinations and paranoia were controlled over several days by changing her medicines and adding a temporary antipsychotic drug therapy. Clearly, the serious lesson was that for Earlene, four medicines together were too much. Each of the drugs had the possibility of causing hallucinations, which she had never had before, but the added effects of all four together caused her to hallucinate and could have resulted in a terrible outcome.

The message for all Parkinson's patients is, before adding a new medicine, always ask your doctor if you can stop or lower the dose of another medicine to avoid compounding side effects.

Controlled-Release Sinemet versus Immediate-Release Sinemet

Controlled-release (CR) Sinemet, a brand of carbidopa/levodopa, differs from the immediate-release form of the drug in that it is absorbed more slowly in the intestines and allows for longer dopamine activity in the brain. The peak dose in the blood occurs about two to two and a half hours after taking it and lasts about six hours, compared to immediate-release Sinemet, which peaks about thirty to forty minutes and lasts about three hours. Therefore, if a patient is having a "wearing off" of the immediate-release Sinemet, changing to the controlled-release form may lessen this problem.

It is important to be aware that some patients do not absorb the controlled-release form consistently and may not seem to benefit with this change. Also, some patients who are taking the CR form may feel much slower in the morning for the first two hours before the dopamine levels peak. Taking a dose of immediate-release Sinemet with the first dose of Sinemet CR can easily prevent morning slow time. For patients who have symptoms of restless legs or who have to get up in the middle of the night to urinate and have trouble moving because of PD, taking a dose of Sinemet CR just before bed can help considerably.

One patient, Barbara, was 80 years old and had had PD for three years. Her daughter Cindy noted that she became much slower an hour and a half before her next dose of immediate-release Sinemet was due. She needed help to get off the couch and had to either use her walker or hold on to her daughter's hands so that she could walk without falling. She was taking one and a half Sinemet IR 25/100 pills at 7 A.M., 11 A.M., 3 P.M., and 7 P.M. By changing to Sinemet CR 50/200 at the same times, she was able to lessen the wearing off so she could get up on her own and walk without help.

General Guidelines

The longer you have Parkinson's disease, the more likely it is that you will be on multiple medications. Although a person might begin with a dopamine agonist, most people with Parkinson's disease will eventually need to also be on carbidopa/levodopa to control the motor symptoms of Parkinson's disease effectively. And ultimately, many patients end up on a dopamine agonist in combination with carbidopa/levodopa and a COMT inhibitor.

Some general rules for using carbidopa/levodopa and the dopamine agonists are listed below:

- Start only one new drug at a time, and observe for a clinical benefit or intolerable side effect.
- Begin with the lowest dose (i.e., Permax 0.05 milligrams, Sinemet 25/100).
- Take your dopamine agonists three times daily, evenly spaced throughout the day, and take your carbidopa/levodopa two to three times a day, and *stick to a strict schedule*. Taking the medication on a regular schedule at set times is extremely important and will lower the risk of having motor fluctuations and allow better control of your Parkinson's disease motor symptoms.
- Avoid taking carbidopa/levodopa close to meals by waiting a half an hour after taking the pill before eating or waiting an hour after eating before taking the pill, in order to allow maximal gastrointestinal absorption. Protein will compete with carbidopa/levodopa and prevent it from getting into the intestines.
- Your doctor should slowly titrate—or adjust—dopamine agonists no faster than doubling the lowest dose every one to two weeks (i.e., Mirapex 0.125 milligrams three times a day in week one, then 0.250 milligrams three times a day in week two or three).
- Your doctor should be aware of the potency differences among the dopamine agonists. For example, 0.5 milligrams of Permax roughly equals 0.5 milligrams of Mirapex and 5.0 milligrams of Parlodel. Requip is much less

potent, and individual doses of 8 to 12 milligrams may be needed before clinical benefit is reached.

- Your doctor may titrate Sinemet by increasing by half of a 25/100 pill with each dose every two weeks (i.e., one Sinemet immediate-release 25/100 pill three times a day in week one, one and a half 25/100 pill three times a day in week three, then two 25/100 pills three times a day in week five).

- No maximal dose exists for the dopamine agonists and Sinemet. The lowest dose that achieves satisfactory clinical benefit while avoiding unacceptable side effects should be chosen.

- If you are having nausea with a dopamine agonist, take it at the beginning of each meal. If you are having nausea with carbidopa/levodopa, ask your doctor to prescribe 25 milligrams of a small orange pill named carbidopa to take with each dose of carbidopa/levodopa. This almost always stops the nausea.

◆ ADJUNCTIVE MEDICATIONS FOR THE TREATMENT OF PARKINSON'S DISEASE

Although carbidopa/levodopa and the dopamine agonists are the most effective medications for the treatment of the motor symptoms of Parkinson's disease, several other classes of medications—including amantadine, the anticholinergics, MAOB inhibitors, and the COMT inhibitors—may be used on their own or in combination with these standard drugs.

Amantadine

Amantadine, which is prescribed by its brand name Symmetrel, is an antiviral agent that has been used to treat the flu, and was found to help Parkinson's patients by reducing tremors, rigidity, and bradykinesia. Although its exact mechanism of action is unknown, it has been proposed that amantadine may act as an N-Methyl-D-aspartate (NMDA) receptor antagonist. These NMDA receptor antagonists may protect dopamine brain cells from toxic damage, while also alleviating some of the symptoms of Parkinson's disease. Amantadine, therefore, may have an added neuroprotective effect, protecting dopamine cells from injury.

Amantadine was one of the first medications used to treat Parkinson's disease and is considered to be a relatively weak drug compared to carbidopa/levodopa and the dopamine agonists, but it clearly does help to reduce Parkinson's disease motor symptoms and recently has been shown to lessen dyskinesia. It is typically given in a dose of 100 to 200 milligrams, two to three times a day.

It can cause side effects similar to those of carbidopa/levodopa and the dopamine agonists, including nausea, vomiting, light-headedness, low blood pressure, anxiety, insomnia, confusion, and hallucinations. A more rare side effect, known as livedo reticularis, involves a purple-red mottled or marble-like appearance of the skin. The medication should be stopped if this or other intolerable side effects occur.

In some patients, amantadine might work initially, but within weeks or months the benefits may stop. But in some patients, amantadine can offer dramatic substantial benefits.

For example, 48-year-old Peter, after eight years of Parkinson's disease, began having an increase in dyskinesia that was difficult to control despite many medication adjustments. He was on Sinemet 25/100 five times a day, taking it every three hours, plus Comtan five times a day, and Permax 1 milligram at 8 A.M., 2 P.M., and 8 P.M. Any decrease in his Sinemet, Permax, or Comtan caused him to become too slow and rigid, and resulted in an increase in "off" time that made it difficult for him to walk, get up out of a chair, and simply move at all. However, with the three medications, he had up to four hours a day of dyskinesia—unpredictable and uncontrollable rapid movements of his arms and legs. Amantadine was added three times a day, and the results were exciting, as Peter reported to his doctor:

> That drug is great—I feel like a new person, I have almost no dyskinesia. Why didn't you put me on it earlier?

Some patients will have a dramatic lessening of dyskinesia similar to Peter's with amantadine, but patients should know that it doesn't happen with everyone and that not everyone can tolerate the medicine without side effects.

Anticholinergics

Like amantadine, the anticholinergics have been around a long time, and in fact were the first medications to be used for the treatment of Parkinson's disease in the 1940s. The commonly prescribed drugs in the United States are trihexyphenidyl (Artane) and benztropine mesylate (Cogentin). These medicines have not been very effective in lessening bradykinesia (slowness), but do clearly help to lessen tremor and muscle rigidity and may reduce excessive drooling. However, they are not as beneficial as carbidopa/levodopa and the dopamine agonists and tend to cause more side effects, which limits their role in the treatment of Parkinson's disease, especially in the elderly patient.

Common side effects include confusion with or without hallucinations, urinary retention, blurry vision, dry mouth, hypotension, and constipation.

Sam was a 56-year-old patient with a relatively rare form of Parkinson's disease, called tremor-predominant type, which features almost no rigidity and bradykinesia, but tremor. In Sam's case, he had fairly constant tremor of his right hand at rest and sometimes with use or while holding a book or newspaper. The tremor did not respond to three different dopamine agonists or low-dose Sinemet, so he was prescribed low doses of Artane—2 milligrams two times a day. Sam had a reaction to the drug.

> Two days after starting it, I woke up in the middle of the night wrestling the floor lamp thinking it was a terrorist. The next day I had a bizarre hallucination: I was covered in black feathers and the ends of my arms and legs were metal, like the Tin Man. It lasted for about twenty minutes, which really scared me, so I stopped it. The next day I was back to my normal self.

While these sorts of reactions are more common in patients older than Sam, unusual reactions to Parkinson's drugs can happen to patients of any age and should always be reported to your doctor.

Selegiline

Selegiline, which is known by brand names Eldepryl and De-prenyl, is a monoamine oxidase (MAO) B inhibitor that can be used with carbidopa/levodopa to reduce motor fluctuations and increase "on" time. It should be prescribed at a 5-milligram dose two times daily, with the first dose taken on waking and the next dose taken not later than 2 P.M., in order to reduce the side effect of insomnia and vivid dreams. Various animal laboratory studies have shown a neuroprotective effect, meaning it prevents dopamine cells from injury and death from toxins, but it has not yet been proven to be a neuroprotective agent in human Parkinson's disease patient studies. The DATATOP study in 1989, which involved 800 mild, early Parkinson's disease patients, showed that selegiline delays the progression of motor symptoms by about nine months, but this again is thought to happen because it enhances carbidopa/levodopa activity to control Parkinson's disease motor symptoms. Overall, selegiline has a limited role in the treatment of Parkinson's disease, as it helps improve motor symptoms only to a small degree, is not proven to slow down Parkinson's disease, and can cause unwanted side effects. Some of the side effects, which are more common in the elderly, include insomnia, nightmares, hallucinations, and more rarely, heartburn, nausea, dizziness, loss of appetite, constipation, and worsened dyskinesia.

One patient, Mark, had been on Eldepryl for twelve years.

It was the first drug I took for PD; I was really young and the doctors thought it might slow my PD down. It did help for the first five years—my tremors were less and I could move better. I am now on Sinemet and

Permax too. I haven't had any side effects from the Eldepryl, so I still want to continue taking it.

Barbara did not have as much luck with the drug and suffered side effects.

When I first took Eldepryl, I felt irritable and hyper and had frightening nightmares . . . I saw dead people chasing me. I stopped it right away and the nightmares stopped.

COMT Inhibitors

The COMT inhibitors are relatively new drugs released in the late 1990s that prevent the breakdown of levodopa and thereby allow more levodopa to enter into the brain. The two available drugs are entacapone (Comtan) and tolcapone (Tasmar). These drugs should be used only with carbidopa/levodopa, and they help to decrease "off" time by one to three hours a day and may allow for a lowering of the total daily dose of carbidopa/levodopa by 10 to 30 percent. Comtan is dosed at 200 milligrams with each dose of carbidopa/levodopa, up to a maximum of eight tablets per day, and Tasmar is dosed at either 100 or 200 milligrams for a maximum of three times a day every eight hours.

It is important to know that the side effects of carbidopa/levodopa (dyskinesia, nausea, confusion, etc.) can occur or increase when a COMT inhibitor is added. The way to prevent this or treat these side effects is to lower the dose of carbidopa/levodopa, rather than stop the COMT inhibitor. Diarrhea occurs in 3 to 4 percent of patients, which can be severe in some cases and occur up to three months after starting the drug. Other side effects include blood in the urine (hematuria) in less than 1 percent of patients.

These drugs can give a dark yellow-orange color to the urine, which is not harmful. It is important not to bite the tablets, however, as the teeth can become stained yellow-orange, and some patients have noted their sweat to stain a similar color on their clothing.

Tasmar, but not Comtan, has also been linked to a very small chance of liver failure; it caused the death of three people with Parkinson's disease in Europe, out of thousands of patients using the drug. Since those reports, Tasmar has been banned for use in Europe and is available for use in the United States, but with strict monitoring of liver function with routine blood testing. If you begin Tasmar, you should have a blood test to check your liver function before starting it and then every two weeks for the first year, followed by less frequent testing after that. If your liver functions become elevated by three times the normal value, the drug should be stopped immediately and your liver function should be closely monitored until it returns to normal.

Richard's story illustrates the importance of frequent testing. Richard had Parkinson's disease for five years, and was taking his Sinemet every two hours because of frequent wearing off. When Tasmar was released, he started on it, after it was shown that he had normal liver function and no history of liver disease. After two weeks of being on Tasmar, he was feeling better, had less wearing off, and he could take his Sinemet every three hours. His liver function was normal until the sixth week, when it jumped to five times the normal value without any warning! Despite this, he felt fine. He was taken off Tasmar, and in five days the liver function returned to normal.

Because of the rare but possible harm to the liver, Tasmar

use has fallen out of favor by doctors and patients, but in some patients, it can improve motor functions and wearing off. Comtan is not as effective as Tasmar, but in some patients may lessen wearing off. The chief benefit, however, is that Comtan is safer, without any risk to the liver.

If you begin one of these medicines, you should watch for a definite reduction in slow time or wearing off within two to three weeks of starting the drug. If no clear benefit occurs, you should stop the COMT inhibitor.

Lucy had "on-off," wearing off, and dyskinesia, and was on several medicines for her Parkinson's disease. After lowering the Sinemet dose and adding Tasmar, she was like a different person.

> I feel like my doctor gave me back five years. It's like a miracle . . . the dyskinesia is almost gone—I went from six hours to only one hour a day—and the Sinemet lasts in between the doses. I am a little slower about a half an hour before the next dose, but not as bad as before.

Donald also had wearing off in between his Sinemet doses, but was concerned about the possible side effects of the Tasmar.

> I would slow down about an hour before the next dose, as if my batteries were running out. It was harder to get up and I felt like I was walking in mud; my legs were heavy. I tried Sinemet CR, but it didn't help and the other drugs made me sick to my stomach. After taking Comtan, I didn't slow down as much. . . . It's made a definite improvement.

General Guidelines

- If you have confusion, hallucinations, or difficulty with memory, review your medication list with your prescribing physician, and if you are taking selegiline (Eldepryl), trihexyphenidyl (Artane), or benztropine (Cogentin), you should be tapered off one drug at a time until your thinking returns to normal.
- You should be on a COMT inhibitor only if you are also taking carbidopa/levodopa. These medications prevent the breakdown of levodopa, allowing more of it to cross into the brain so that it can work better to lessen the motor symptoms of Parkinson's disease.
- Selegiline (Eldepryl) was originally thought to slow the progression of Parkinson's disease; however, later studies have not supported this and it has a limited role in treatment.
- The anticholinergics should be used sparingly in the treatment of Parkinson's disease, due to their increased risk of significant side effects, but in patients with severe tremor that does not respond to carbidopa/levodopa or the dopamine agonists, they may be very helpful in reducing the tremor.
- Amantadine (Symmetrel), once thought to be a relatively weak drug, has made a comeback as an adjunctive medication and in some patients may dramatically lessen dyskinesia. Some Parkinson's disease specialists use this as a first-line drug as in theory it might be neuroprotective, meaning it might protect dopamine brain cells from dying.

Botulinum Toxin

Botulinum toxin is a synthetic drug made from the bacteria that causes botulism, and is available in the United States in two forms, type A (Botox), which is the older of the two and has been studied for a variety of uses in Parkinson's disease, and type B (Myobloc). Botox has been used for treatment of a variety of spastic muscle disorders, including hemi-facial spasm, blepharospasm, and torticollis.

It works by preventing the release of the chemical acetylcholine from the nerve at the neuromuscular junction. This chemical is needed to allow muscles to normally contract. When botulinum toxin is injected with a needle through the skin directly into the muscle, it causes the muscle to weaken and lessens the spasms or rigidity in the muscle. It takes three to five days after the injection before it begins to work, and the results last about two to three months before it wears off, requiring repeat injections.

The use of botulinum toxin in the treatment of Parkinson's disease is limited. It has been formally studied for the treatment of tremors by injecting it into the muscles of the arm that cause the tremor, but the results were not very promising. The botulinum toxin weakened hand muscles and reduced functional use of the limb, without any substantial reduction in tremors. The drug has seemed more promising when treating selected leg or neck muscles, especially if the patient has only a few overactive muscles. Botulinum toxin may be helpful with foot dystonia, which involves cramping and painful turning in of the foot that can make walking even more difficult for the Parkinson's disease patient. It has also been used to treat excessive drooling by injecting the toxin directly into the salivary glands. It is considered to be a very safe drug in that it does not interact with other medications. The main side effect is weakening of the muscles that are injected.

Additional Medications for Difficult-to-Treat Tremor

Some patients with Parkinson's disease may have tremor that is severe and does not get better with any of the standard medications listed above. Other medications to consider trying that might help to lesson the tremors include mirtazapine (Remeron), gabapentin (Neurontin), topiramate (Topamax), benzodiazepines (Xanax, Ativan, Klonopin), beta-blockers such as propanolol (Inderal), and atypical antipsychotics such as clozapine (Clozaril).

◈ WARNINGS AND INTERACTIONS

A good rule of thumb when starting any new medication is to first consult your physician and review all of the medications you are taking. Next, ask your pharmacist to review all of your medications for possible drug interactions or combined side effects. The more medications you are taking, the more room there is for error and for problems to occur. Routinely review your medications and ask each of your prescribing physicians why you are taking each medication that he or she is prescribing and then ask whether you really need it. If it is not helping you or if it is causing side effects, you should probably stop taking it.

For instance, you might have been on medication for high blood pressure for the past five years and then be diagnosed with Parkinson's disease and start a dopamine agonist such as Permax, and then note that your blood pressure is too low and that you feel light-headed or dizzy when you stand up. The

Permax may be lowering your blood pressure, and you may need to lower the dose of the high-blood-pressure medication or even stop it altogether.

With carbidopa/levodopa, antacid medications such as cimetidine (Tagamet), ranitidine (Zantac), and famotidine (Pepcid) should be taken two hours apart from carbidopa/levodopa to allow proper absorption.

Dopamine-blocking drugs that reduce dopamine activity should be avoided in persons with Parkinson's disease, as they will likely worsen rigidity, tremor, and bradykinesia and counteract the benefits of the dopamine-stimulating medications. These include strong D2 receptor blockers, the antipsychotic medications typically used to treat schizophrenia or mania such as haloperidol (Haldol) and chlorpromazine (Thorazine). Some of the medications used to treat nausea also block dopamine activity and can also worsen Parkinson's disease motor symptoms. These drugs include prochlorperazine (Compazine), promethazine (Phenergan), and metclopramide (Reglan).

Selegiline can interact with some of the SSRIs—the antidepressant medications that prevent the uptake of a chemical in the brain called serotonin—and cause what is called a serotinergic crisis. This is extremely rare, but can occur and be very dangerous in that the person can develop high blood pressure, excessive sweating, diarrhea, vomiting, confusion, headache, high heart rate, chest pain, and high body temperature requiring hospitalization. Some of these SSRI antidepressants are fluoxetine (Prozac), sertraline (Zoloft), paroxetine (Paxil), fluvoxamine (Luvox), and citralopram (Celexa). This does not mean if you are taking selegiline that you cannot take an SSRI, but you should be aware of this rare possibility.

In addition, selegiline should never be given with meperidine (Demerol) because of the very rare possibility of a dangerous and potentially fatal change in the heart rhythm. Demerol is commonly used to treat pain after surgery, so if you are going to have planned surgery and you are taking selegiline, be sure to talk to your surgeon. It is generally recommended that you stop the selegiline at least two weeks before surgery and that you make sure that Demerol is listed as an allergy in your hospital chart so that it is not given to you.

A common misconception among pharmacists is that a patient on selegiline needs to be on a special tyramine-free diet to avoid the risk of high blood pressure (this is true with MAO type A, but not type B, inhibitors; selegiline is type B). This is not true as long as one does not exceed the daily dose of 10 milligrams total (5 milligrams two times a day) of selegiline. Many over-the-counter cold medications include a warning not to take them if you have Parkinson's disease. This again is based on false belief that selegiline is unsafe when combined with some of these medicines.

❖ MANAGING MOTOR COMPLICATIONS

If you are having wearing off or dyskinesias, there are some possible changes to your medicines that you may wish to discuss with your doctor.

Possible treatments for wearing off (worsening Parkinson's disease motor symptoms before the next dose of medicine) include the following:

- Use Sinemet CR (controlled release) or Sinemet ER (extended release).
- Add a dopamine agonist.

- Add a COMT inhibitor to Sinemet (immediate release, CR form, or ER form).
- Take Sinemet more frequently.

Treatment of dyskinesia (irregular, writhing movements of limbs, head, or trunk) may include the following:

- Change from Sinemet CR or ER to immediate-release form.
- Lower the dose of Sinemet and shorten the time in between doses.
- Add a dopamine agonist.
- Add amantadine.
- Try liquid Sinemet.

Liquid Sinemet

For patients who have extreme "on-off" or cannot tolerate a half a dose of Sinemet 25/100 because of dyskinesia, preparing liquid Sinemet and taking it every one hour at a lower dose can provide relief from dyskinesia and lessen off time. Liquid Sinemet is not commercially available in a liquid form and needs to be prepared by your pharmacist or made at home as follows:

1. Purchase a one-liter plastic container with a lid, a cooler bag, and a smaller 25-to-50-milliliter measuring cup.
2. Mix the following in the container:

   - Sinemet 10/100 or 25/100 immediate release (do not use controlled release, CR), 10 pills
   - Vitamin C crystals or crushed tablet, 2 grams
   - Tap water, 1 liter

3. Gently shake the mixture, and then keep refrigerated, out of sunlight.

This formula makes a 1-milligram-per-1-milliliter dose and allows for greater fine-tuning of the dose of Sinemet than does the pill form.

Before taking the liquid Sinemet, gently shake the container. While your doctor will prescribe the dosage for you, a typical starting dose would be 60 to 70 milliliters for the first dose of the day, followed by 30 to 40 milliliters every hour throughout the waking hours of the day. The dose can be adjusted up or down by 5 to 10 milliliters as needed. If you are too slow, then increase the hourly dose by 5 to 10 milliliters, and if you are too fast with dyskinesia, decrease the hourly dose by 5 to 10 milliliters. A fresh batch should be made every one to two days.

The most important thing to realize in managing medications for the treatment of Parkinson's disease is that each person is completely different from the next and will respond differently to different medications. You and your physician will need to continually reassess the medications you are taking and make changes to find the formula that works best for you over the long course of your life.

❖ MEDICATION WARNINGS

Some of the drugs that you need to be particularly careful about taking if you have Parkinson's disease include the following:

Antipsychotic Drugs

Chlorpromazine (Thorazine)
Chlorprothixene (Taractan)
Fluphenazine (Prolixin)
Haloperidol (Haldol)
Loxapine HCL (Loxitane)
Mesoridazine besylate (Serentil)
Molindone (Moban)
Olanzapine (Zyprexa)
Perphenazine (Trilafon)
Risperidone (Risperdal)
Thioridazine (Mellaril)
Thiothixene (Navane)
Trifluoperazine (Stelazine)

Antidepressants

Perphenazine and amitriptyline (Triavil)
Phenelzine (Nardil)
Tranylcypromine (Parnate)

Antivomiting Drugs

Droperidol (Inapsine)
Metoclopramide (Reglan)
Prochlorperazine (Compazine)
Thiethylperazine (Torecan)

Medications for the Treatment of Parkinson's Disease

Key:

First line—These are the first drugs most physicians will consider.
Second line—These are drugs that are considered when first line drugs are not effective enough to sufficiently control disabling symptoms.

Third line—These are drugs that are considered by the physician when first and second line drugs are failing to control symptoms.

bid—twice a day

tid—three times a day

Medication	Starting Dose (mg)	Potential Side Effects	When This Drug Is Used
Carbidopa/Levodopa			
Carbidopa/ levodopa (Sinemet, Atamet)	25/100 bid/tid	hypotension, nausea, confusion, dyskinesia	First line, or add to dopamine agonists
Carbidopa/ levodopa controlled release (Sinemet CR, Sinemet ER)	50/200 bid	hypotension, nausea, confusion, dyskinesia	First line, or add to dopamine agonists
Dopamine Agonists			
Bromocriptine (Parlodel)	2.5 tid	hypotension, nausea, livedo reticularis, confusion, edema	First line, or add to L-dopa
Pergolide (Permax)	0.05-0.25 tid	same as bromocriptine	First line, or add to L-dopa
Pramipexole (Mirapex)	0.125 tid	nausea, hypotension, sleep attacks, sedation, hallucinations	First line or add to L-dopa

Medication	Starting Dose (mg)	Potential Side Effects	When This Drug Is Used
Ropinirole (Requip)	0.25 tid	nausea, hypotension, sleep attacks, sedation	First line or add to L-dopa
Amantadine Hydrochloride (Symmetrel)	100 bid/tid	same as bromocriptine	Second line/motor fluctuations
Anticholinergics Benztropine mesylate (Cogentin)	0.5 bid	confusion, hallucinations, blurry vision, dry mouth, urinary retention, nausea	Second line/ refractory tremor
Trihexyphenidyl HCL (Artane)	1-2 bid	same as Cogentin	same as Cogentin
Monoamine oxidase B inhibitors			
Selegiline (Eldepryl)	5 bid (no titration, this is max dose)	agitation, insomnia, vivid dreams, hallucinations	Third line, little role for PD
Catecholamine-o-methyltransferase (COMT) Inhibitors			
Entacapone (Comtan)	200 with each dose L-dopa, max 8/d	hematuria, diarrhea, levodopa S. E.	Add to L-dopa Second/wearing off
Tolcapone (Tasmar)	100 tid	same as Entacapone, hepatotoxicity (liver monitoring required)	Add to L-dopa Third/motor fluctuations

Chapter 6

Surgical Treatments for Parkinson's Disease

Great thanks are due to Nature for putting into the life of each being so much healing power.

—*Johann Wolfgang von Goethe*

◆ SOME HISTORY

From the 1940s through the 1960s, before the discovery of effective medications for the treatment of Parkinson's disease, surgery of the brain was the primary treatment for Parkinson's disease. In fact, tens of thousands of brain surgeries for Parkinson's disease—known as thalamotomies and pallidotomies—were performed in Europe and the United States. Some clinical benefits occurred, with reduction in tremors and rigidity, but they were not long-lasting effects and the surgical techniques back then were much riskier, with more permanent side effects and with a mortality rate as high as 12 percent.

After levodopa was discovered by Dr. George Cotzias in 1967, the use of these surgical procedures declined dramatically, as the drug was a safer and less invasive alternative. In the past two decades, however, a renewed interest in surgical treatment of Parkinson's disease has taken place. The main reason for this is that patients are living much longer with Parkinson's disease, thanks to the benefits of medication. The longer one lives with Parkinson's disease, however, the more likely the person is to develop disabling symptoms that the medication may not effectively control. Patients may have a wearing-off effect, such that the medication does not last long enough and they need to take more frequent doses of the medicine. In extreme cases, patients may have to take a pill every one to two hours in order to function. Patients may also experience dose failures, when the medication just doesn't seem to work at all.

Other patients may develop dyskinesias—involuntary writhing, often rapid, dancelike movements of the limbs, trunk, head, and sometimes face—which are thought to be a long-term complication from the medications for Parkinson's disease. These movements can be even more disabling than the tremors and slowed movements of Parkinson's disease.

Some patients may alternate throughout the day between the hyperkinetic state of dyskinesia and slowed, "off" time, where they have difficulty moving. These patients may be fast one hour and slow the next.

Another important reason for the increase in surgical treatments for Parkinson's disease in the last twenty years is that medical technology has dramatically improved. The once risky surgery is much safer than it was in the 1940s and 1950s. New equipment and techniques have been developed and are more effective in treating some of these chronic motor problems.

◆ AN INTRODUCTION TO SURGERY

The main problem in the electrical pathway in the brain of a person with Parkinson's disease is that the final motor circuit from the thalamus to the motor cortex is inhibited, or not working at full capacity. In order to enhance and restore positive electrical signals to stimulate the motor cortex, so that a patient can have better movement, the pathways must be adjusted, much the way an electrician would fix an electrical short. This can be done in one of two ways: by creating a lesion or hole (similar to a small stroke) or by inserting a metal wire called an electrode, which is then turned on to electrically stimulate the motor circuit.

Three main types of surgical treatments have been used for the treatment of Parkinson's disease. These include the following:

- **Lesioning:** This involves creating a small hole ("otomy") in the brain. Depending upon where the hole is put, a different name is given to the procedure. For example, a lesion in the thalamus is called a thalamotomy, and a lesion in the globus pallidus is called a pallidotomy. (Lesioning of the subthalamic nucleus—subthalamotomy—has not been found to be an effective therapy.)

- **Electrical Stimulation:** This involves placing a thin wire with an electrode at the end into the brain and then turning on the electrode to stimulate the brain motor pathways. The electrode may be placed at three different places in the brain: the thalamus, globus pallidus, or subthalamic nucleus. This procedure is called deep brain stimulation, or DBS for short.

- **Tissue Transplantation:** This involves taking some type of living tissue (from an aborted human fetus, from the fetus of an animal such as a pig, or from the patient) that contains dopamine cells and directly putting them into the brain of a patient with Parkinson's disease. The results of tissue transplantation have not been particularly successful, however, and these procedures are considered to be experimental in comparison to the other types of surgery.

Whatever surgery is performed, the goal is to improve motor function in patients who have advanced disease and are not responding to medications.

Surgery is usually performed only on one side of the brain in the case of lesioning techniques, while some patients may benefit from staged (separated by time) bilateral DBS.

The left side of the brain controls motor function on the right side of the body and vice versa. This is critical to understand, because since surgery for Parkinson's disease is typically done on one side of the brain, the benefits will be seen on the opposite side of the body. For instance, if a patient had tremor, stiffness, and slowness that were worse on the right side, then surgery would be performed on the left side of the brain, to improve the right-body function. After such a surgery, there would not typically be an improvement of the body's motor function on the left side.

Note from Dr. Jill: Lesions and Electrical Stimulation

When you put a lesion in the globus pallidus, you're effectively causing what's known as "disinhibition." By putting a lesion in the brain, we block—or inhibit—a malfunctioning pathway and allow the final circuit to be turned back on, resulting in the patient's being able to move efficiently and effectively.

Similarly, by placing an electrode at the same point and stimulating it at a high frequency, the final motor pathway is turned back on, allowing for more improved movement. When using the same electrode and stimulating at a low frequency (i.e., 50 hertz), however, the motor pathway is less efficient, and symptoms can sometimes even worsen.

How is it that a lesion can make something better, a high-frequency electrode can make it better, yet a lower-frequency electrode in the same place can make it worse? We truly don't understand the detailed mechanism of why these surgical procedures work. What we are attempting to do is learn to talk to the brain and understood its language.

However, while we've merely stumbled onto this information and don't fully understand it, the good news is, in the vast majority of patients, it truly works!

❖ ARE YOU A CANDIDATE FOR SURGERY?

Surgery is not for everyone; in fact, most Parkinson's disease patients do not need brain surgery. However, if you are relatively young (or older and in good physical health), have advanced Parkinson's disease, and your medication isn't helping, then you may want to consider surgery. Patients who have disabling dyskinesia may also benefit greatly from surgery. According to Dr. Rajish Pahwa, director of the NPF Parkinson Center of Excellence at Kansas University, "Approximately 15 to 20 percent of patients with PD can benefit from surgery."

Before considering surgery, however, it is extremely important that you see a neurologist who specializes in Parkinson's disease, so that all drug and treatment options can be properly tried, over a sufficient amount of time. This is a very critical point. Before subjecting yourself to invasive surgery, it's essential that you consult with a Parkinson's specialist, because such an expert may be able to adjust your medication and improve your motor symptoms, thereby avoiding surgery.

Steven, a 56-year-old married attorney and father of four, was diagnosed with Parkinson's disease at age 48 and had tremors and marked slowness or "off" time, when it was almost impossible to move and do anything. He had considerable improvement after an adjustment to his medications, which included carbidopa/levodopa. However, after several years, he developed severe, disabling dyskinesia. Lowering the doses of his medication could reduce his dyskinesia, but this resulted in the return of marked "off" time. After two years of riding a roller coaster of alternating dyskinesia and "off" time, he was considering deep brain stimulation therapy. Shortly after that, a new medication for Parkinson's became available, tolcapone. Steven started the medicine. A few weeks later, his physician barely recognized him. When before, he would march in with arms and legs flailing due to the dyskinesia, after a few weeks on the new drug, he walked in like anyone without Parkinson's disease.

Indeed, he did not need surgery after all. This dramatic improvement is not common, but it does occur and many patients can realize significant improvement after modifying their medications under the direction of a Parkinson's disease expert.

The decision to have surgery should be made by you together with your family and your neurologist. What type of procedure to have will depend upon what your symptoms are, and this decision should be largely left up to the Parkinson's specialist, although there does seem to be a trend toward deep brain stimulation (DBS) of the subthalamic nucleus as the preferred procedure among Parkinson's disease surgical specialists. Details about each procedure, including clinical indications, benefits, and complications, are outlined below. It is extremely important that you find a center that has modern stereotactic equipment, as well as a neurosurgeon who is experienced in the use of this equipment and skilled in these techniques. You may have to rely on your Parkinson's specialist to guide you in this search.

Take your time in finding the right surgeon and center. This is not emergency surgery; it is elective and should be done on your timetable—if and when you need it and are ready to have it. Get a second or third opinion, shop around, meet the neurosurgeon and ask him or her how many procedures he or she has done and what his or her results are. Talk to patients who have had the same procedure, and ask for literature to read and videotapes to watch about the surgery. Good surgical centers for Parkinson's disease should provide you with these resources.

◆ TYPES OF SURGERY

Thalamotomy

Thalamotomy involves using a heat-sensitive probe to create a small hole in the thalamus of the brain. This technique is very effective at reducing tremor in Parkinson's disease, as well as essential tremor, by as much as 90 percent. Long-term benefit— lasting up to ten years—has been reported in patients who have had a thalamotomy. However, many patients do not experience a marked reduction in rigidity and bradykinesia with this procedure. Therefore, the only candidates considered optimal for a thalamotomy would be patients with severe essential tremor that is unresponsive to medications or patients with a rare form of Parkinson's disease, called tremor-predominant Parkinson's disease, in which the patient has little or no rigidity and bradykinesia but has a disabling tremor that is not controlled by medication.

The mortality rate for the surgery is, on average, less than 1 percent, and is mainly due to brain hemorrhage. Possible complications from the surgery include weakness or numbness on the opposite side of the body, partial visual loss, seizures, gait difficulty, slurred speech, and infection. Complications are fairly uncommon, however, and occur only in a small percentage of patients. In the case of thalamotomy and pallidotomy, the neurological symptoms may be permanent, as they result from brain tissue being destroyed during the procedure. Bilateral thalamotomy—lesioning of both the right and left thalamus—is associated with a 30 percent risk of severe difficulty with speaking and swallowing, and since most experts agree that the risks far outweigh the benefits, this surgery is usually not performed.

Pallidotomy

Pallidotomy is similar to thalamotomy, except that the lesion is placed in a different part of the brain, the globus pallidus. Pallidotomy is by far the more commonly performed lesioning surgery. Only recently have clinical studies begun to document the effects of this procedure. Current data suggest that patients may benefit from this procedure, with a reduction in tremor, rigidity, bradykinesia, and off time by 15 to 50 percent at four months, and even up to four years after surgery. Some patients with tremor were shown to have a reduction of up to 75 percent, when using microelectrode recording.

The number of patients followed over a long term is small,

and thus the long-term benefit of pallidotomy is not truly known. Some patients will have an initial dramatic improvement of their motor function after the surgery, only to lose that benefit six weeks, six months, or a year after the surgery. Other patients, however, have enjoyed a more-than-five-year persistent benefit from the surgery.

Dyskinesia seems to be the most improved symptom, with a marked reduction by as much as 80 to 90 percent. Patients whose main difficulty was with their walking and balance did not have marked improvement in their walking.

The ideal candidate for pallidotomy is a patient with disabling Parkinson's disease that is not controlled with medications, or a patient who has disabling dyskinesia, but no dementia or difficulty with mental processing.

The mortality rate for this surgery has declined from 12 percent in the 1950s to less than 1 percent. Serious side effects occur in 1 to 8 percent of patients and may include weakness on the opposite side of the body, partial loss of vision, slurry or muffled speech, depression, difficulty swallowing, and seizures. There is some inherent risk of error based on anatomy and variability in the brains of patients, such that even with the best technology, a lesion can be placed incorrectly, or slightly off of the desired target. This is usually the cause of permanent neurological symptoms. If this occurs, however, many times these symptoms improve slowly and steadily over months or a year, just as in the case of a stroke. Any infection that may follow is usually treatable, and the seizures that rarely occur after the surgery are usually readily controlled with antiseizure medicines.

Bilateral pallidotomy has been associated with impaired mental processing as well as slurred speech and difficulty swallowing, and, like thalamotomy, it is rarely recommended.

Ralph is 72 years old and has had Parkinson's disease for twelve years. Two years ago he had a pallidotomy on the right side of his brain.

I had gotten so slow that it was hard to do anything without my wife's help. When we increased the medicine, I was so wiggly with dyskinesia that I couldn't control my arms and legs—I would jump around and my wife had to feed me and help me get dressed and to take a bath. I was on five different medications for the Parkinson's, and I was either too slow or too wiggly. I felt like a puppet—like someone else was controlling my body. At first I was afraid of having the surgery, but then I thought, "How much worse could this get?" I had to try something. I talked to a couple of patients that had had DBS and pallidotomy and visited the center three hours away and met the surgeon and neurologist and a month later had the surgery. The surgery took about five hours. I could tell the difference almost right away—I could move my left arm and leg in the operating room. Once I started taking my medicine for the Parkinson's disease, I could move like before, but with much less dyskinesia on the right side of my body and none on the left side at all. I think I got a little better the first month after the surgery. I still have to take a lot of medicine, mostly for the right side of my body, my left arm and leg feel almost normal and I hardly ever wiggle, so it was a definite success.

At age 58, Jeanette had a pallidotomy on the left side of her brain after having Parkinson's disease for fifteen years.

It was like a miracle—my right arm and leg didn't shake anymore and they weren't as stiff and slow. I was so happy, then only eight weeks after the surgery I started shaking like before and got slower and stiffer, and it was almost like I hadn't had the surgery at all. That was over six years ago. No one could understand how or why it didn't last. Luckily, I didn't have any bad side effects, but had I known this would have happened, I wouldn't have had the pallidotomy. The doctors tell me I can have DBS surgery, but I'm not ready to try it. I'll just stick to my medication for now.

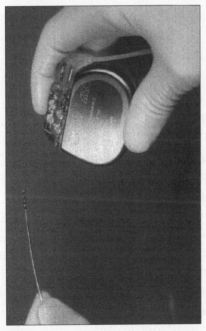

Figure 4a. An electrode used in deep brain stimulation. The electrode is connected to a battery pack that is implanted in the chest (Figure 4b, next page). (Courtesy of Medtronic, Inc.)

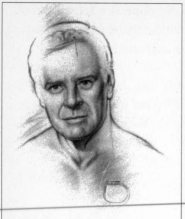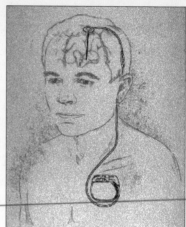

Figure 4b. Courtesy Medtronic Inc.

Deep Brain Stimulation (DBS)

Deep brain stimulation (DBS) is a relatively new technique pioneered by Dr. Alim-Louis Benabid in France in the late 1980s. It involves placing a metal electrode into the brain at the thalamus, globus pallidus, or subthalamic nucleus sites, connecting the electrode to a battery source, and continuously stimulating the brain at a high frequency (100 to 180 hertz).

DBS of the thalamus results in a marked reduction of tremor in 92 percent of Parkinson's disease patients, with results lasting up to eight years or more. However, similar to thalamotomy, the other motor symptoms of Parkinson's disease—rigidity and bradykinesia—are not greatly reduced by thalamic DBS. Therefore, DBS of the thalamus is seldom performed for the treatment of Parkinson's disease, except in the case of tremor-predominant Parkinson's disease not controlled by medication.

DBS of the subthalamic nucleus is typically done on one

side of the brain, and it can also be done as a second surgery on the other side of the brain at a later date. Very few centers recommend having bilateral DBS at the same time, as a single procedure, however.

DBS of the subthalamic nucleus has shown great promise, with reports of an 80 percent reduction in tremor, according to the Unified Parkinson's Disease Rating Scale (UPDRS) tremor rating, as well as a 65 percent reduction in rigidity, a 51 percent reduction in bradykinesia, and an 80 to 90 percent reduction in dyskinesia.

Bilateral DBS has been shown to be very effective in reducing the motor symptoms of Parkinson's disease, without the risks of impaired mental functioning, swallowing, and speaking found in bilateral thalamotomy and pallidotomy.

There are reports that some patients who have had bilateral subthalamic nucleus DBS are able to function independently without medications for Parkinson's disease. Most patients after DBS to the subthalamic nucleus are able to reduce their daily dose of medication for Parkinson's disease by 30 to 50 percent.

In research reported in the journal *Neurology* in late 2001, deep brain stimulation was found to increase the amount of "on" time by 29 percent. Even in "off" time, motor function was improved by 38 percent. The patients studied were able to complete a walking test 13 percent faster when the stimulator device was on. Patients also had a 23 percent improvement in a finger-tapping test that measures bradykinesia, the slowness in initiating movement.

A study reported in the *New England Journal of Medicine* compared bilateral DBS of the subthalamic nucleus to bilateral DBS of the globus pallidus sites in 134 patients with Parkinson's disease. This study found that patients who received bilateral DBS to both sites had beneficial effects six months after surgery, with an increase in "on" time without dyskinesia from 27 to 74 percent in the subthalamic nucleus group and from 28 to 64 percent in the globus pallidus group. Nine patients had major adverse reactions—seven had intracranial hemorrhage and two had infection requiring that the electrodes be removed. While there are still not enough patients and long-term data to know how long these benefits may last, the example of DBS to the thalamus—where patients have had continued reduction of tremor for over ten years—suggests similar promising results.

Deep brain stimulation is not without risks and hassles. Unlike pallidotomy, which is a onetime procedure, DBS requires that the electrodes be programmed and the battery pack or pulse generator—which is inserted under the skin of the chest—changed every two to five years. These procedures can be done under local anesthesia. In some cases, the electrodes have had to be repositioned or removed because of malfunction, improper positioning, hemorrhage, or infection.

Mortality rates for DBS, however, are extremely low, with only one reported case of death in North America. Serious side effects are seen in 2 percent of patients, and these can be permanent neurological deficits such as difficulty opening eyelids, weakness and numbness, and strokelike symptoms. Temporary, reversible complications include seizures, confusion, scalp or wound infection, electrode scalp erosion, numbness of the face or hand, and dyskinesia.

Karen, who was only 32 when she was diagnosed, had the deep brain stimulation procedure.

I was diagnosed twelve years ago and had the surgery four years ago. It's made all the difference: I feel younger and healthier and have been able to return to work as a teacher part-time and can take care of myself and my daughter July, who's now 15 years old and demands more attention than when she was three. The surgery gave me back my life.

Jerry was diagnosed at age 38, and only three years later, he started having severe, debilitating dyskinesia that was so bad that he described it as making life not worth living.

I found a doctor that specialized in Parkinson's and for one year we tried all different combinations of medication: We tried Tasmar, adding more dopamine agonists and lowering the Sinemet dose, we even tried low doses of liquid Sinemet, and we added Amantadine. You name it, we did it, and nothing really made a big enough difference. So at age 48 I had an electrode put into the right side of my brain. Even though they didn't turn on the electrode until a month after surgery, I felt better the next day. Four months after the first surgery, I had a second electrode put into the left brain. Now it's over a year since my last surgery and I am 80 percent improved. No more uncontrolled movements. I can do everything by myself; before the surgery my wife had to help me all the time. When asked if I would recommend this to someone like me, I say, "In a New York minute." Life is worth living again because of the DBS surgery.

Sherry had a rare form of tremor-predominant Parkinson's disease that caused her right arm and leg to shake almost all of the time, but she had very little slowness or muscle rigidity.

She was almost never without tremors, whether at rest or when she used her hand.

After eight years of shaking all the time and trying over ten different drugs that didn't help, I decided to have the surgery. The doctors said I could have an electrode or a small hole [thalamotomy] put into my thalamus on the left side of my brain and that my tremors had an 80 to 90 percent chance of calming down. I decided to have the electrode because I thought the doctors could adjust it to better control the tremors. The surgery was great—I had almost no tremors in the operating room when they turned on the electrode! Two weeks later, I had a horrible headache and started vomiting and felt like I was drunk. I called my neurologist and was told to come to the emergency room right away. A brain scan showed a big blood clot on the outside of my brain under my skull [a subdural hematoma]. I was taken right away to the operating room and the surgeon removed the blood clot. I was okay but very frightened. After that, the tremors got worse again and with three months of programming they didn't get better. The surgeons thought I should have the electrode removed because it wasn't working and probably got moved during the second surgery to take out the blood clot. So I had the electrode taken out and the battery pack removed, and at the same time they put the little holes in my thalamus. Three total surgeries and two years later I have about 60 percent less tremor and no side effects or problems. I definitely think it was worth having the surgery, I just wish I had chosen the thalamotomy first.

Gamma Knife Radiosurgery

One procedure similar to thalamotomy and pallidotomy is gamma knife radiosurgery. In this procedure, an external beam of radiation is aimed at either the thalamus or globus pallidus, to create a small lesion similar to the hole created during a thalamotomy or a pallidotomy, without having to directly cut or touch the brain. This procedure has not been a widely accepted and applied therapy for Parkinson's disease to date, as it is not as effective in reducing the motor symptoms of Parkinson's disease as pallidotomy and DBS. It may be considered as an option by some patients, in that it is a less invasive surgical procedure. However, because the safety of it and long-term benefits are not proven, it is not something most Parkinson's disease patients should have. As with pallidotomy and DBS, accurately hitting the target seems to be the key to success.

Pallidotomy or DBS

Although we do not have good studies and results comparing lesioning and stimulating techniques, and more studies are needed, the general opinion is that DBS is more beneficial and has less risk of serious side effects than a pallidotomy. Because the electrodes can be adjusted—turned on and off, amplitude changed, frequency and pulse width adjusted—the benefits and side effects can be controlled to some degree. With pallidotomy, it is a onetime procedure, and if a bad result such as weakness or numbness occurs, it will likely be permanent.

Some patients, however, are better candidates for a pallidotomy rather than a DBS. Patients who do not live near a medical center that can program the electrodes, or who do not want the electrode in their brain, or do not want to have the battery periodically changed, or are on strong blood thinners such as Coumadin may be much better suited for a pallidotomy. Age does not really seem to be a factor when deciding between the two procedures, except that an older person may be able to tolerate pallidotomy because it is a quicker procedure and doesn't involve the intense programming of the electrodes. It really is a decision that needs to be made in consultation with your neurologist and neurosurgeon, who can review the details, risks, and benefits of each surgery with you. The majority of surgical centers that do these surgeries today perform more DBS procedures than pallidotomies.

Can More Than One Type of Surgery Be Done on the Same Patient?

The answer is yes, there are patients who have had a pallidotomy on one side and then had DBS on the other or same side at the subthalamic nucleus. Others have had a thalamotomy on one side and DBS of the subthalamic nucleus or the globus pallidus on the opposite side.

The general rule is not to place an electrode where a lesion has already been made, but it appears effective to place an electrode at one site if a lesion has been done at a different site. The patients who have had multiple or combination lesion therapy and DBS seem to benefit most from the DBS, although we truly do not have large enough numbers of reported similar cases to draw any meaningful conclusions about multiple surgeries for Parkinson's disease.

Rita had advanced Parkinson's disease that affected both sides of her body. She suffered from marked slowness and tremors and rigidity as well as uncontrollable dyskinesia. After a long battle that left her almost completely dependent upon her husband, Bob, she had a pallidotomy on the left side of her brain. It was almost immediately successful in lessening the dyskinesia on the right side of her body, and she had very little tremor and speedier movement on the right side. However, six weeks after the surgery, she developed worse tremors and dyskinesia on the left side of her body. Rita said it was as if "the Parkinson's just switched sides."

Two years later Rita decided to have DBS surgery on the right side to improve the left body function. At that time, she could barely do anything without help from Bob, she was either too slow or tremulous or had too much dyskinesia, and sometimes she would have both violent tremors on the left side and dyskinesia on the right side of her body at the same time.

Two months after the DBS surgery, Bob was pleased with the results.

> It wasn't a cure and we didn't expect that; all we wanted was some improvement. She has very little dyskinesia, maybe a mild amount or one to two hours a day, whereas before the surgery she would have five to six hours in a row of bad writhing of her whole body. She couldn't do anything during those times; I had to feed her like a baby and carry her if she wanted to move out of the bed. She couldn't walk without help from me. Now she can walk slowly with a cane, and she can feed herself and dress herself. She still needs help during her slower times, maybe about three hours out of a fourteen-hour day.

Rita also considered her DBS a success.

The DBS gave me back a lot of my independence—I feel like a human being again. Bob can have more of a life. He's a saint for all he's done for me. Now we can relax a little—Bob doesn't have to stay with me all the time, and he's golfing again. We can actually go out to a movie or to dinner with our friends. We used to just hide inside our house; our social life was going to see the doctor. I'm so happy I had the surgery; I'm learning how to live again. I had almost forgotten what it was to be happy.

Tissue Transplantation

Since the early 1980s, when adrenal gland transplantation was first performed, tissues that are rich in dopamine have been transplanted into the brains of patients suffering from advanced Parkinson's disease. This procedure involved taking part of the patient's own adrenal gland and then putting it directly into the brain. Adrenal transplantation was not proven to be successful, and given its risks, it was quickly abandoned.

Shortly afterward, human fetal brain cell transplants were introduced, and over two hundred Parkinson's disease patients in several different countries had the procedure by the early 1990s. Results have been varied, mostly due to the variety of techniques. Some patients have enjoyed a dramatic improvement, while others had little benefit. In some cases, patients had serious side effects and even died.

One of the most recent studies had to be stopped due to an unacceptably high rate of disabling dyskinesia that occurred in patients who had the fetal transplants. In fact, some of these patients required a pallidotomy to improve the dyskinesia that resulted from the tissue transplantation surgery. Those results, along with the ongoing ethical debate over using aborted human fetal tissue, and the higher cost of the procedure, have made tissue transplantation less popular, and it is considered experimental at best.

The ethical concerns over fetal tissue have also focused interest on use of pig fetal brain cells. These cells have also been studied and transplanted into human Parkinson's disease brains, but like the human fetal transplants, these procedures have not had great success. Other research currently under way is evaluating the transplantation of human cells from the retina.

Overall, while tissue transplantation is being studied and explored (see chapter 11), and more effective procedures may be available for human studies in the near future, this type of surgery is currently experimental and is not considered to be a proven treatment for Parkinson's disease.

◆ THE DO'S AND DON'TS OF SURGERY FOR PARKINSON'S DISEASE

Do . . .

- Do consider surgery if you have disabling advanced Parkinson's disease that in the past was responsive to carbidopa/levodopa, but has become less effective over several years.
- Do consider surgery if you have disabling dyskinesia that is not corrected by medication changes.
- Do find a Parkinson's disease specialist to discuss the possibility of surgery and to be sure all medication changes that might improve the Parkinson's disease symptoms have been tried.

- Do bring someone else to every appointment to have a second pair of eyes and ears to ask questions and hear the doctor's input.
- Do get written and video educational materials about the types of surgery and the risks and benefits.
- Do talk to several people who have had the surgical procedure you are considering.
- Do get a second or third opinion before proceeding with surgery.
- Do meet the neurosurgeon well before deciding whether to have the surgery, and bring written questions with you about the surgery and about what will happen during the procedure and after. Ask the surgeon about his or her credentials and the success and complication rates of the patients at his or her center. Most centers that do brain surgery for Parkinson's will do a minimum of two surgeries a month, and many do two a week.
- Do ask about whether to take your medication on the day of surgery (most centers will ask the patient not to take the medicines for Parkinson's disease the day of surgery). Review all of your medications, including vitamins and herbs, with the surgeon, as some may increase the risk of hemorrhage, such as vitamin E, ginkgo, aspirin, Coumadin, etc., and may need to be stopped a week or more before surgery.
- Do know when to go and whom to see to have the electrodes programmed if you have an electrode (DBS) placed in your brain. (The neurologist or the neurology nurse typically does this one month after surgery.)
- Do know where and when to have your stitches taken out.

- Do know whom to call if you have a complication after surgery, and keep the phone number handy (give a copy of this to your spouse or family member).
- Do know the financial cost of the procedure and whether your health insurance covers the costs or not. (One DBS can cost up to $35,000, and one pallidotomy can cost up to $20,000.)

Don't . . .

- Don't have any type of surgery if you do not want to for whatever reason.
- Don't consider surgery for Parkinson's disease if it is mild or manageable.
- Don't have DBS surgery if you have a cardiac pacemaker. (You can have a lesioning procedure, however.)
- Don't consider surgery for Parkinson's disease if you have other serious health problems and the doctors think the surgery could be risky (such as severe heart or lung disease).
- Don't consider surgery if you have dementia (difficulty with memory) or impaired mental health (severe depression or hallucinations).
- Don't have a bilateral (right and left brain) pallidotomy or thalamotomy—the risks of slurred speech, difficulty swallowing, and impaired memory or thinking far outweigh the benefits.

◈ THE ACTUAL SURGERY

Presurgery Tests

If you have decided on surgery, you will typically undergo some or all of the following tests and evaluations before the actual surgery date. This will usually occur weeks to months before surgery.

- MRI of the brain
- Chest X-ray
- Blood tests (CBC, chemistry panel, pregnancy test if female and of childbearing age, PT/PTT to evaluate bleeding times)
- EKG 12 lead, to evaluate heart rhythm
- Complete history and physical examination, by a neurologist and neurosurgeon
- UPDRS motor rating in an "off" state without medicine for Parkinson's disease and in an "on" state with medication's best control of Parkinson's disease symptoms (by the neurologist). This may be videotaped. (If it is taped, be sure you sign a consent form, so that you can indicate whether or not you will allow your tape to be used for educational purposes.)
- Evaluation of your thinking, including neuropsychiatric tests to rule out dementia
- Review of all your medications, and a discussion of whether any need to be stopped before surgery, such as blood thinners

Once you have a surgery date, be sure to ask your physician ahead of time for a mild sedative to help you sleep the night before. Most people will be very nervous the night before surgery, and a good night's sleep will make your surgery day better. If you are traveling from out of town to the surgical center, be sure to arrive ahead of time by one full day—or even two if possible—to allow enough rest and for any unforeseen delays in your travel plans. Many hospitals will offer discount rates on hotels close to the hospital for patients and their families. The night before surgery, you should not eat anything after midnight.

The Day of Surgery

You should not take your medicine for Parkinson's disease after midnight the night before surgery or on the morning of your surgery. Other medications—such as for high blood pressure, diabetes, etc.—usually can be taken on an empty stomach; however, you should review this with the surgeon prior to your surgery. Most centers have the patient check in very early, around 6 or 7 A.M. the day of surgery. Shortly after arriving at the hospital admitting desk, you should be greeted by one of the surgery nurses and given a place to change into a hospital gown.

Typically, the next step is that the neurosurgeon will place the special stereotactic frame on your scalp. The area for surgery will be shaved. (Bring a hat or purchase a wig ahead of time, as it may take several months or more for your hair to grow back, depending on the length.) After shaving, you will have the skin of your head cleaned and be given local anesthesia to lessen the pain from the screws of the frame, which will penetrate the skin around your head. Despite having local anesthesia, you may feel pressure and some discomfort while it is being applied. The process of having the frame applied will take anywhere from a half an hour to an hour. You will remain in this frame all morning and during the entire surgery, until the lesion or electrode has been placed. The frame helps the surgeon find the right target. Special computer software fuses the pictures from the MRI and CT scan into one image, to allow precise localization of the place in the brain to place either a lesion or an electrode.

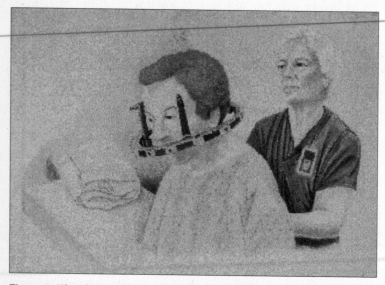

Figure 5. The electrode used for deep brain stimulation is inserted with the help of a special stereotactic frame. (Courtesy of Medtronic, Inc.)

After the frame is applied, you will have a CT scan done of your brain while the frame is in place. After the brain scan, you will be taken to the operating room, where there will be between four and six people, including nurses, doctors, and surgical assistants.

You will be awake throughout the entire procedure of placing the lesion—thalamotomy or pallidotomy—or the electrode (deep brain stimulator). If you have a lesioning technique, you will not need any general anesthesia. If you have an electrode placed, you will have brief general anesthesia for the time when the connecting wire and pulse generator—a battery pack—are inserted under the skin of the neck and chest wall. This process usually takes about forty to sixty minutes. The overall time you will be in surgery is anywhere from four to eight hours.

The surgery will begin with a local anesthetic to the scalp. Next, the surgeon will use a drill to make a small (less than the size of a quarter) circular hole in your skull. This will not hurt, but the sound of the drill may be unsettling. The anesthesiologist may give you a mild sedative in the beginning to help calm you for the surgery.

Once the hole is made in the skull, the surgeon will place a probe into the brain, using the targets from the computer brain scan. This may take several hours. You should not feel any pain, but you may feel a tingling sensation around your mouth or in your hand. You should report anything you feel during the entire surgery, and especially during the probe placement, to the surgeon. Your observations may actually help them in finding the right target. The doctors will listen to the brain cells with a special electrode (either a semi-macroelectrode or microelectrode) to assist in target location. When the surgeon thinks the probe is in the correct spot, you will be asked to move your arms and legs, and one of the doctors (usually the neurologist) will check your muscle tone and the speed of your movements and observe for tremors. In the case of DBS, the brain electrode will actually be turned on and adjusted to see if tremor, rigidity, and bradykinesia improve.

Sally describes the middle of her surgery:

The doctors asked me to lift up my right arm, and I couldn't do it (I didn't have any medicine that morning like they said and I was so slow and stiff). Then they turned on the electrode and I almost hit the frame with my hand, it was so light, like a feather. I couldn't believe it. I knew they were in the right spot.

When the correct target has been found, you will have several small holes placed in the brain if you are having a lesioning technique, or you will have a permanent electrode placed and left at the target site if you are having DBS. Either a small plastic cap or special hard gel foam will be inserted to fill the hole in the skull. Stitches will be placed in the scalp (usually eight to ten), and in the case of DBS, there will also be stitches in the neck behind the ear and on the chest wall over the battery pack.

After the surgery is done, you will go to a postoperative holding area for about two hours, where nurses will check your blood pressure and give you pain medicine. You will then go to a regular hospital room. You should be able to take all of your regular medications, including the ones for Parkinson's, after surgery. Be sure to bring your medicines from home in case the hospital doesn't have all of them. Your doctor can write an order so that you can keep them at the bedside to be sure you get them on time.

Most patients can go home the day after surgery. Some centers will check another brain scan after DBS surgery to look for the electrode placement.

After Surgery

Whether you have had a pallidotomy or DBS, you may not feel very different immediately after surgery. Some patients, however, notice a marked improvement in Parkinson's disease tremors, rigidity, bradykinesia, or dyskinesia right away. Others, more commonly DBS patients, may experience a delayed improvement in Parkinson's disease symptoms up to one to two months after the surgery, so don't be disappointed if you do not feel an immediate benefit.

Patients who have a pallidotomy or thalamotomy do not need any special procedures. They should see the neurosurgeon and neurologist within a month of surgery for follow-up, and frequently during the first six months after surgery, to evaluate the effects of the surgery.

In the case of DBS, the electrode is typically not turned on until one month after surgery. The brain seems to need a month to recover from the surgery, and if the electrodes are programmed before one month, the benefit stops and they will need to be reprogrammed. As noted before, however, some patients do experience some improvement in the period between surgery and when the electrodes are turned on. You'll need to return for the turning on and adjustment of the electrodes about one month after surgery, and likely several times after that—every two to three weeks or so—until the correct setting is found that controls the Parkinson's disease motor symptoms without any side effects.

These programming sessions will take between one to two hours and are usually done at the neurologist's office with a specially trained nurse. A handheld electrical device is placed over the battery pack under your chest, and the electrode settings (frequency, amplitude, pulse width) are adjusted (figure

3). You may be asked to come to the appointment without having taken your medicine for Parkinson's disease and then take it after arrival to check for control of your symptoms in an "off" and "on" state.

Side effects that can occur after DBS with the stimulator on include

- Tingling (paresthesias) in the hand or face
- Weakness (paresis) in arm or leg or face
- Slurry speech (dysarthria)
- Dizziness or light-headedness
- A jolting or shocklike sensation
- Rapid jerking movements of the arm or leg (ballismus)

Adjustment of the electrodes can almost always lessen or stop these side effects if they occur.

Andy talks about his trials and tribulations with DBS surgery.

The decision to have the surgery was easy. I knew I needed it and I researched it enough to know it was the right thing to do. The Parkinson's disease after sixteen years was just too tough to take—I was either too slow or had bad dyskinesia. Three months ago I had an electrode put into my left brain. The surgery itself was no big deal; it's the three months after surgery that have been the problem. First, I got an infection where the battery was put under the skin of my chest—the scar where the stitches were got hot and red. So I started taking antibiotics and thought that was that. But a week later I felt a big bump where the scar was. The infection had gotten worse and become an abscess [a collection of pus]. The surgeon had to cut my skin and drain it and then put the stitches back in again. I had to take two more weeks of antibiotics. A month after surgery the infection was gone. Then we turned on the electrode and I had better movement on the right side of my body and less dyskinesia, but I get a tingling and tremor in my tongue and tingling in my right hand and foot when the electrode is on. I've had the electrodes adjusted every two weeks for the last month and a half, and I don't think it has made a big enough improvement. Right now if you ask me if it was worth having the surgery, I would say no. I was expecting to be a lot better than I am.

Some key points regarding after-surgery care:

- Gradually return to your normal activities, but avoid any strenuous physical activity the first month.
- If you have an electrode in place, avoid contact sports or any activity that could cause the electrode and battery pack to be moved or damaged.
- Have an appointment to get your stitches removed seven to ten days after surgery. In the meantime, keep the stitches and wound sites clean by washing around them, not on them, with warm soapy water, then dry. Do not scratch or pick. Watch for infection of the wound sites (if the area becomes red, swollen, tender, or hot or has liquid draining from it, call your doctor immediately. You may need to take antibiotics and possibly have the area surgically drained).
- Resume all of your medications immediately after surgery, according to your regular dosage and schedule. (The neu-

rologists will not likely adjust the Parkinson's disease medicine before one month after surgery.)

- Resume your regular diet.
- Have a list of doctors' phone numbers to call in your wallet and give the same list to at least one other person, in case of an unforeseen problem after surgery (i.e., infection, seizure, confusion).

For patients who have an electrode (DBS) implant, there are some additional items to be aware of regarding use of electrical devices:

- You will have two small magnets that you can hold up to your battery pack or pulse generator, and by counting "One one thousand, two two thousand" while holding it over the skin, you can turn it either on or off. (Always keep one with you.)
- Your electrode should remain on at all times, however. The only time it should be turned off is by your physician, who may turn it off for testing.
- If you believe your electrode is causing unwanted side effects—such as tingling of the arm or face or jerking of the arm, leg, or face—contact the physician for evaluation, but do not turn off the electrode.
- You can use cellular phones and regular kitchen appliances and computers.
- You will have a slight bulge on the chest wall and a three-to-five-inch incision scar where the pulse generator is placed. This will not be visible under most clothing, but will be readily seen if it is not covered.
- The theft detectors in stores can cause you to feel uncomfortable stimulation and can turn off the electrode. If you

feel uncomfortable when approaching a store, walk in the middle of the detector.

- Large refrigerators and freezers can turn your electrode on or off.
- You may set off the airport detectors, so keep the identification card that comes with your magnets in your wallet, to explain that you have an electrical device in your body.
- You should not have an MRI, as it could affect the function of the electrode and battery, except under the supervision of the neurologist or neurosurgeon.
- DO NOT use dithermy or ultrasound.
- Some patients cannot tell if the electrode is working or not. They may want to use a new device that can be placed on the chest wall over the battery (pulse generator) and that lights up if the electrode is turned on.

❖ DAVID'S STORY

David, who was diagnosed at age 48, suffered increasingly worsening dyskinesia after six years on carbidopa/levodopa. His symptoms became so severe that he could not drive. Says David:

> I had spells where when I was sitting in a chair I would slide out of the chair and onto the floor and would begin flailing and thrashing. I had that happen at work, at church, in stores . . . just about everyplace I went I would be having dyskinesia. I knew it was what hell was like. A person who went to hell would get the kind of dyskinesia that I had.

David became interested in pallidotomy as a possible treatment for his dyskinesia. He was evaluated and scheduled for a pallidotomy. David describes his experience:

The morning of surgery finally came. I could take no Parkinson's disease medication after the evening meal. I ate no breakfast that morning. We arrived at the hospital at 6:00 A.M. I was escorted to my room, where I was given a hospital gown and told to put it on and take my street clothes off. Then I was put on a gurney and was taken to where they put the stereotactic frame on my head. The only part that hurt at all was when they screwed it into my ears while they set the other screws in position. Then they screwed the frame to the gurney so I could not move my head.

David had a few starts and stops that day, and the stereotactic frame was removed, and then put on again, and David was finally wheeled to the OR for surgery. He continues his story:

I was told that I must stay awake for the entire procedure. The first thing that the doctor did was take measurements of every part of the frame. Next they shaved two little patches just above my hairline. Then the doctor took a drill—the one that the doctor used was stainless steel, but it was hand-powered. He proceeded to drill a small hole in my head. After that, there was discussion of calculations from MRI pictures and coordinates on the frame. They continued to ask me questions during the surgery; they often had me count from ten down. They did a lot of tinkering inside my head until they got to the target. First he touched the target with a probe and said, "Raise your right leg." I did so. But it was much easier than it had been. When he was sure that he was at the target, he turned the probe on and heated it to 185 degrees and burned a small hole in my globus pallidus. After one stitch to close the wound, the frame was removed from my head and I was wheeled to a recovery area.

David did not get out of bed until the next morning. He got up and dressed himself with no difficulty. His wife came, and they checked out of the hospital at 10 A.M. Says David:

Hours later, I noticed that there was no dyskinesia of any kind. I was thrilled. I had just had my life given back to me. Before, even when I was not having the violent dyskinesia, I was moving all the time if I had taken Sinemet. I was either off or I was dyskinetic. There was no middle ground. But that was all behind me now. At first I did occasionally have a little dyskinesia, but nothing like before. And as time went on, I had less and less dyskinesia. I thought that until my brain recovered from surgery, I would not experience all the benefits of the pallidotomy. That seemed to hold true—I continued to improve during the first six months after my surgery. The really big thing was the lack of dyskinesia. Now it has been six years since that day. I am still without dyskinesia.

◈ WHEN SURGERY DOESN'T WORK

Some patients do not have a marked improvement after lesioning or DBS surgery. In the case of pallidotomy, if it is not beneficial, there is unfortunately little if anything that can be done. It is important to understand that this is a real possibility before making the decision to have surgery. If you are not willing to accept this possibility, then avoid this type of surgery. In the case of DBS, remember that it may take many sessions of programming the electrodes over several months before the full benefit is achieved. If, however, six months to a year after either type of surgery no benefit is observed, then it should be concluded that the surgery was not successful. If this occurs with DBS surgery, you should consider having the electrode removed or repositioned.

◈ CONCLUSION

Surgical treatment is a therapy to seriously consider for people with advanced or disabling Parkinson's disease that is not well controlled with the available medications. Surgery is not without some risk, and is not 100 percent guaranteed to work, but overall, it can be very beneficial in the majority of patients who have these procedures. It is estimated that 20 percent of all persons with Parkinson's disease currently meet criteria for surgical treatments, and this number may increase in the next decade.

Many patients who have lesioning surgery or deep brain stimulation have found that the procedures had a profound positive impact, reversing and lessening Parkinson's disease motor symptoms and motor fluctuations.

Part III

ALTERNATIVE AND COMPLEMENTARY THERAPIES

Chapter 7

Complementary and Mind-Body Approaches

The essential philosophic quest in the world is for integration—which is to say, the need to bring together rational philosophy, scientific knowledge, personal experience, and direct observation into an organic whole.

—Norman Cousins

This chapter first explores some general ideas behind complementary medicine, then describes how to choose alternative treatments and practitioners, and finally introduces several of the most promising types of alternative medicine for Parkinson's disease patients. A comprehensive look at herbal and nutritional approaches to Parkinson's disease is featured in chapter 8.

❖ COMPLEMENTARY OR ALTERNATIVE MEDICINE

If you're reading this book, you're already a believer in one aspect of complementary medicine—a patient's involvement in his or her own health care. Becoming more educated about and involved in your own health is a fundamental part of the concept of complementary or alternative medicine.

What Is Complementary Medicine?

But what is complementary medicine, and what could it possibly offer to people with Parkinson's disease? Complementary medicine can go by a variety of names—some people refer to it as alternative medicine. Berkeley, California, holistic practitioner Dr. Stephen Langer says, however, "I hate the term 'alternative medicine,' because if it's right, it's not alternative!" Dr. Langer touches upon a valid point. Referring to a type of medicine as "alternative" isn't even really an accurate concept. The word sets up the idea that what are deemed "alternative" approaches—such as herbal treatments, acupuncture, Ayurveda, mind-body medicine, and other modalities—present an either/or decision to patients. Most of these approaches can actually work best as complements to what are considered conventional approaches. When approaches are combined, working with a carefully selected combination of the best of complementary and conventional treatments, this is truly "holistic" or "integrative" medicine at its best.

Whatever terminology you use, the basic idea is to view the person and his or her condition as all part of a whole, a system. This differs from the conventional Western medicine approach, which is to focus solely on the disease and focus all treatment specifically on the disease—or in this case, the symptoms, because there are no conventional "cures" for Parkinson's disease itself. In contrast, complementary medicine looks at the causes and the nutritional and environmental factors that may aggravate or trigger disease in general and Parkinson's in particular. It considers the nutritional deficiencies that worsen symptoms or speed onset. Complementary medicine looks at the important role of emotions, mood, and stress on health and symptoms, and sees disease as a disequilibrium and imbalance in body, mind, and spirit, not just a constellation of symptoms that warrant treatment.

Researching Options

If you're not already a dedicated fan of complementary medicine, before you launch in, there are some questions you will want to ask yourself:

- Why do I want to try complementary medicine?
- What do I expect from the process and experience?

To answer these questions, it's important to research the available options, so that you can begin to decide which modalities or approaches (for example, meditation, or yoga, or herbs) to pursue. Or, you may decide that you'd rather pursue treatment via a particular medical system, such as Traditional Chinese Medicine or Ayurveda, where one practitioner will direct your treatment within the guidelines of that medical tradition. Or, you may wish to find a holistic M.D. or naturopathic practitioner who will assess your case and recommend particular alternative therapies from among a variety of choices.

To decide on your options, it's important to start by becoming more informed. This book can be a starting point in helping identify some of the complementary therapies that may work well with your treatment program. Two other books can be of particular help in learning more about alternatives, and are highly recommended:

- *Alternative Medicine: The Definitive Guide,* edited by Burton Goldberg (Future Medicine, 1998), weighs in at more than 1,100 pages and is considered the "Bible of alternative medicine." Featuring the input of more than four hundred doctors, including naturopaths, Doctors of Oriental Medicine, and other alternative experts, this book covers many conditions and symptoms, including Parkinson's, and is an excellent resource for learning more about many therapies.

- *Prescription for Nutritional Healing,* by James Balch, M.D., and Phyllis Balch (Avery Penguin Putnam, 2000), is a 776-page essential reference for alternative medicine. The third edition of this book goes through basics of nutrition, vitamins, minerals, herbs, and supplements and their impact on 250 health conditions and symptoms.

As for choosing from among the many options, holistic healer, Reiki practitioner, and health educator Phylameana lila Desy has these additional thoughts:

> Today there are so many treatment choices. I recommend my clients try a variety of methods. I suggest they pay attention not only to how their physical body reacts to these methods but to how their emotional, mental, and spiritual bodies align with the treatment. If a person feels a treatment is bizarre or silly, they may be willing to give it a try, but in reality, they are not truly trusting that it will result in a cure. This untrusting "thought-form" may actually create a barrier between sickness and wellness. Healing touch, Reiki, massage therapy, acupuncture, meditation, herbology, aromatherapy, visualization, and homeopathy are a few of the healing options that are more frequently sought out by people with chronic disease.

One question that is particularly important to raise is whether or not you are keeping your primary care physician or neurologist informed about your interest in or treatment using complementary and alternative medicine. It's extremely important to do so. One study in 2000, published in the journal *Neurology,* found that vitamins, herbs, massage, and acupuncture are commonly used as alternative therapies for Parkinson's disease, and as many as 40 percent of patients used at least one form of alternative medicine. Less than half of the patients, however, consulted their physician. Since many herbs and vitamins can interact with medication, and since complementary techniques can have an important role in the overall picture of your Parkinson's treatment, it's essential that you keep your primary physician informed.

Finally, the last and most important question you need to ask yourself is whether you are prepared to commit yourself to a complementary or alternative therapy. Most of these sorts of treatments involve much more than taking a pill several times a day, and require you to become a truly active participant in your own wellness. Alternative therapies rarely offer a quick fix. You need commitment and patience. Some holistic and complementary approaches aren't easy to follow. You may need to completely overhaul your diet and give up sugar or bread products—completely changing the way you eat. Or you'll need to organize and take dozens of herbal preparations a day, or make regular visits to a physical therapist or other practitioner.

Incorporating Complementary Treatments

If you are determined to incorporate complementary medicine into your treatment program, the first step is to avoid the temptation to self-treat. It has become very common for people to read articles or books, or hear advice from other patients in person or online, and then to immediately start taking herbs and vitamins or making dramatic changes in their diet, without the guidance and supervision of an expert. Parkinson's disease is a complicated condition, and your day-to-day functioning depends on the appropriate treatments—both conventional and alternative. A misstep—even something as simple as taking the wrong herb or vitamin—can dramatically affect how you feel and function, so you simply can't afford to not have professional advice guiding your treatment. So, above all, don't try to choose the right program of vitamins, herbs, and supplements yourself.

The next step is to find reputable alternative practitioners who are recommended by your physician, trusted health advisors, or other patients. If there are licensing or certifications associated with the particular alternative therapy you're choosing, it's always wise to select a practitioner who has the appropriate credentials. For example, you want an herbalist who is a member of the American Herbalists Guild or another credentialing organization—not someone who is selling supplements via multilevel marketing programs and labels himself or herself as an "herbal consultant."

If you're not familiar with the form of complementary medicine or the practitioner, you might want to have an initial meeting, during which you can explore the topic in greater depth. In that meeting, ask about the theory and approach behind this particular modality or treatment, and what specifically is involved in the treatment.

It's also useful to ask about the practitioner's own experience and background for this type of complementary medicine approach. In particular, you'll want to ask how familiar the practitioner is with Parkinson's disease, what his or her typical approaches and success rates are, and even if there are other patients you can speak with to find out more.

Time frames for treatments are critical to discuss. For some people, the longer time frame for treatment involved in some complementary or alternative therapies may be unacceptable, so it's essential to have a sense of what to expect, timewise. For example, "You can expect this herbal treatment to help with fatigue in from six to twelve weeks" means that you will not expect to see improvements after two days or two weeks and will have more realistic expectations.

Finally, costs should be discussed—both practitioner fees and any supplements or other treatments that may be necessary. While most complementary and alternative practitioners—like their conventional counterparts—are honest, there are occasionally practitioners who excessively mark up the cost of supplements, who attempt to sell numerous unnecessary supplements or devices, or who require costly, extensive, and sometimes unnecessary testing, including hair, saliva, and urine analyses as part of their standard treatment. Discussing costs up front will help you weed out the rare unscrupulous practitioner you might encounter.

❖ TRADITIONAL CHINESE MEDICINE

Traditional Chinese Medicine (TCM) is a complete system of medicine that originated thousands of years ago in China.

In TCM, a person is in optimal health when there is free and balanced flow of *qi*. Qi (which is also sometimes written as *chi,* and is pronounced "chee") is the TCM term for vital energy or life force, which is channeled through the various meridians of the body. Many TCM treatments are focused on directing qi to preserve or restore health and balance. In addition to qi, TCM relies on the concept of yin and yang, the interdependent opposites, representing different organs and health aspects. TCM diagnostic techniques include observation, listening, questioning, and palpation, including feeling special pulse qualities and sensitivity of body parts.

TCM treatments include diet, exercises such as t'ai chi and the Qi Gong breathing, herbal preparations, acupuncture, acupressure massage, physical therapy, and moxibustion, which involves the use of heat at specific energy points on the body—either applied directly or to the acupuncture needles—as a way to add energy.

Perhaps the most well-known Chinese treatment, however, is acupuncture. Acupuncture works by accessing invisible internal systems of meridians or channels that conduct qi, or energy. These meridians flow throughout the body, connecting organs and organ systems and surfacing on the body in over six hundred points, known as accupoints. In acupuncture, very thin, fine needles are inserted at the different accupoints to balance, restore, and regulate the body's energy.

According to holistic practitioner Barbara Maddoux, a Doctor of Oriental Medicine and R.N.,

> Some of the benefits of acupuncture include pain relief, improvement of fatigue, strengthening of the immune system, ridding the body of toxins, and reducing the muscle spasms and tremor associated with Parkinson's disease.

Acupuncture has been well studied and proven to be effective for a variety of problems. In 1997, the National Institutes of Health sponsored the Consensus Development Conference on Acupuncture, which found that pain from musculoskeletal conditions and certain postoperative pain and nausea were successfully treatable with acupuncture. In late 1998, a University of Arizona study also found acupuncture an aid in treatment for depression.

While scientists may not understand the concept of qi or how acupuncture works, it's clear that it does work for many symptoms and conditions. In the United States, acupuncture has become an increasingly established practice, both as part of TCM and even more so on its own. Americans make an estimated nine to twelve million visits to acupuncturists annually, and some three thousand conventionally trained U.S. physicians also practice acupuncture.

While there are only a few published studies that look at the benefits of acupuncture for Parkinson's disease patients, those studies have shown that there are specific physical changes that occur in response to acupuncture treatments. According to some TCM practitioners and acupuncturists, the stiff and sore muscles and the imbalance of posture and walking experienced by many Parkinson's patients may be alleviated by an acupuncture treatment that focuses on encouraging the flow of energy or on addressing the tremors and the hardening of the muscles directly.

TCM and Parkinson's

TCM practitioners attribute Parkinson's disease to problems that give rise to "Liver Wind," which causes tremor and affects the muscles and ligaments system. In TCM theory, "Liver" refers not only to the organ but to the associated meridian— or energy channel—and controls coordination and smooth body movements. According to Dr. Maddoux, with a combination of acupuncture and Chinese herbal formulas, Parkinson's disease can be controlled and its progression slowed, but not completely cured. The sooner the treatment is started after onset, the better the outcome.

According to Dr. Maddoux, TCM offers a very specific explanation for Parkinson's:

> *The Original Theory of Medicine,* written in the Ming Dynasty, says tremors may be caused by: deficient original qi, which allows pathogenic factors in the channels so that blood cannot nourish the sinews or channels; deficient qi unable to attract fluids and blood toward sinews and channels to nourish them; deficient fluids and blood not nourishing the sinews; and Phlegm-Fire obstructing the channels and sinews so that fluids and blood cannot nourish them. In all cases, though there are many different causes, there is a deficiency of fluids and blood not nourishing sinews and channels.

Dr. Maddoux explains that TCM identifies three different categories of imbalances that are consistent with Western definitions of Parkinson's disease: Qi and Blood Deficiency, Phlegm-Fire Agitating Wind, and Kidney and Liver Yin Deficiency.

QI AND BLOOD DEFICIENCY

Typically, deficiency is caused by emotional stress, and strong emotions such as anger, resentment, and frustration appear to be connected to the rise of Liver Yang, leading to Liver Wind over time. Some of the clinical signs a practitioner looks for include limb tremor over time, a staring expression or gaze, limb cramps, avoidance or dislike of speaking, and sallowness.

Moving can become difficult, with balance and coordination problems, walking difficulties, and dizziness. Vision may become blurred, and patients may sweat excessively, particularly with exertion or movement. The tongue, an important indicator in TCM, may appear to be pale and swollen, and teeth marks may be evident. Pulse in such patients is typically normal. To treat this imbalance, according to Dr. Maddoux,

> practitioners perform acupuncture, and also recommend specific Chinese herbal formulas that tonify qi, nourish and move blood, extinguish wind and expel wind from the channels.

PHLEGM-FIRE AGITATING WIND

This particular type of imbalance is frequently due to diet, in particular, eating too many greasy, fried, or sweet foods. These types of foods cause the formation of phlegm. In time, Fire combines with the Phlegm, especially if the person regularly drinks alcoholic beverages. On its own, Phlegm-Fire is not considered a direct cause of Parkinson's disease, but when associated with Liver Wind, which it often is in old people, it can trigger the condition. In this imbalance, phlegm blocks the energy channels and prevents fluids from nourishing them, which then results in the tremor.

A TCM practitioner looks for a patient who is overweight, has a staring look, avoids exercise, and has a feeling of heaviness in the chest. Such patients frequently present with a dry mouth, yellowish phlegm, and a red tongue with a sticky yellow coating. In these patients, the neck and back may feel stiff, a tremor may be evident, and patients may suffer from insomnia and sweating. Typically, the pulse is wiry and rapid.

Treatment focuses on resolving phlegm, clearing heat, extinguishing wind, and invigorating the connecting channels. Herbal formulas tonify the spleen, resolve phlegm, and subdue Liver Wind.

KIDNEY AND LIVER YIN DEFICIENCY

This imbalance is usually due to working long hours, without getting enough rest, over long periods of time. Working night or graveyard shifts can also put the body out of sync with Mother Nature and deplete and weaken the kidneys. Liver Yin and Liver Blood then fail to moisten the sinews. This dryness combined with the Liver Wind leads to tremors.

According to Dr. Maddoux, practitioners look for

> a slender frame, feeling dizzy, ringing in the ears, difficulty sleeping, insomnia, dream-disturbed sleep, headaches, night-sweating, feeling of restlessness, sore knees and back, neck stiffness, tremors and cramps in the head, jaw, and limb.

Practitioners also look for a red, uncoated tongue and a fine, rapid pulse.

Treatment focuses on nourishing Yin, extinguishing wind, invigorating the connecting channels, and subduing Liver Wind. According to Dr. Maddoux, the best results are obtained from Qi and Blood Deficiency treatment, and second best from Phlegm-Fire.

Choosing a TCM Practitioner

When choosing a TCM practitioner, be sure to see someone who is licensed and certified. For complete TCM treatment, you'll want to find a Doctor of Oriental Medicine (D.O.M.).

For someone who performs acupuncture, top certification is from the American Academy of Medical Acupuncture (AAMA). Acupuncturists who are not M.D.s can receive credentials known as a Diplomate in Acupuncture (Dipl.Ac.). They may be called Licensed Acupuncturist (L.Ac. or Lic.Ac.), Registered Acupuncturist (R.Ac.), Certified Acupuncturist (C.A.), Acupuncturist, or Doctor of Acupuncture (D.Ac.). Each state has its own specific requirements for practice of acupuncture. Be sure your TCM practitioner or acupuncturist is nationally certified from an organization like the National Certification Commission for Acupuncture and Oriental Medicine (NCCAOM).

Forceless Spontaneous Response and the Parkinson's Recovery Project

An interesting program specifically addressing Parkinson's disease with a combination of acupuncture and Asian medicine was developed by Janice Walton-Hadlock and is disseminated by the Parkinson's Recovery Project. Walton-Hadlock has developed a system of Yin-type TuiNa—which includes a form of Chinese medical massage and acupuncture—that is known as FSR (forceless spontaneous response). FSR is reported to result in varying levels of relief from Parkinson's disease symptoms, including tremor, rigidity, decreased dyskinesia, and problems with balance and circulation. The program is reported to work regardless of the stage of the disease, and Walton-Hadlock reports an ability to reduce the amount of conventional medication taken.

A group of patients who are following Walton-Hadlock's FSR treatment have an online support group to exchange information. For more information or to join the group, visit their information and signup page, http://groups.yahoo.com/group/PDrecoverers/.

In the support group's archives, there are a variety of stories from patients, who reported that even as early as after ten sessions of FSR, levels of medication were able to be reduced by more than half, and that symptoms such as rigidity and tremor were greatly reduced or even disappeared. Another woman reported that her 78-year-old father, who had had Parkinson's for ten years and was wheelchair-bound, was able to walk on his own again with no help after the second treatment, with continued improvements after each treatment.

Walton-Hadlock's detailed manuals for both practitioners and patients are available free online, in Adobe PDF format:

- Recovery from Parkinson's Disease: A Practitioner's Handbook
  http://www.pdtreatment.com/publications/pd_prac_v5.pdf
- Appendix—Practitioner's Handbook
  http://www.pdtreatment.com/publications/pd_app_v5.pdf
- Recovery from Parkinson's Disease: A Patient's Handbook
  http://www.pdtreatment.com/publications/pd_pat_v5.pdf

Information about the treatment and the Parkinson's Recovery Project is available at their Web site, http://www.pdtreatment.com. This group's objectives include disseminating information regarding Parkinson's disease treatments that use techniques of Asian medicine, researching efficient treatment plans, and creating a database of patient information.

◈ AYURVEDIC MEDICINE

Ayurveda (pronounced "Ah-your-vay-duh") has been the traditional medicine of India for more than five thousand years and is perhaps the oldest medical system in existence. *Ayurveda* is a Sanskrit word that means "science of life" or "life knowledge," and is based on the premise that the body naturally seeks harmony and balance. In Ayurveda, disease represents emotional imbalance, unhealthy lifestyle, toxins in the body, and most particularly, imbalances in what are known as doshas. Doshas are different regulatory systems—*vata* (movement), *pitta* (heat, metabolism, and energy), and *kapha* (physical structure and fluid balance)—that govern different aspects of health. According to Ayurveda, proper balancing of the doshas is accomplished through food and diet, herbs, meditation and breathing, massage, and even yoga poses to ensure that energy is flowing. In this way, the concept of balance and energy makes Ayurveda similar to Chinese medicine.

Some naturopaths or homeopaths offer aspects of Ayurvedic treatment or incorporate Ayurvedic herbal preparations as part of their treatments. There are also purely Ayurvedic practitioners. Typically, Ayurvedic practitioners make a diagnosis by asking detailed questions to assess your dominant dosha, and taking ayurvedic pulses, among other diagnostic tools.

Ayurveda and Parkinson's Disease

Ancient Ayurvedic texts provided a description of Parkinson's disease, which is referred to as "Kampavata." Most promising for Parkinson's patients, however, is an Ayurvedic treatment that uses a substance known as *Mucuna pruriens*. This remedy has been shown to help Parkinson's disease sufferers.

Mucuna pruriens is a twinelike plant, native to India, that has triangle-shaped leaves, purple flowers, and curved pods. The pods cause intense itching if they come in contact with human skin. In the 1930s, scientists isolated levodopa from the beans of *Mucuna pruriens,* decades before the discovery of levodopa as a Parkinson's disease treatment. In the 1960s, after levodopa was introduced as the primary treatment for Parkinson's disease, a widespread analysis of more than one thousand species of 135 different families of plants found that only plants in the *Mucuna* family had sufficient amounts of levodopa to make it commercially viable as a drug.

In the United States, one of the leaders of Ayurvedic studies for Parkinson's disease is Dr. Bela Manyam, a professor of neurology at the Scott and White Clinic in Temple, Texas, which is part of the Texas A & M Medical School. Dr. Banyam's center, which is also a National Parkinson Foundation Center of Excellence, conducted studies using a powder made from the whole bean of *Mucuna pruriens*.

Mucuna pruriens is a legume (bean) and, in addition to high levels of natural levodopa, has high levels of vitamin E. The high-fiber content of *Mucuna pruriens* also makes it a laxative that helps digestion and reduces constipation, which is frequently found in Parkinson's patients. *Mucuna pruriens* may also contain other as yet unidentified ingredients that help Parkinson's patients.

Dr. Manyam studied sixty early, nonadvanced Parkinson's patients at approximately Stage 2.5 on the 1–5 Hoehn and Yahr staging system. The research found that all sixty patients who took *Mucuna pruriens* had improvement of almost one entire stage. It's also thought that, with more study, naturally occurring compounds in the plant may offer safer and improved treatments for Parkinson's disease.

Remember that use of Ayurvedic medicines such as *Mucuna pruriens* is best done under the guidance of a trained practitioner. In addition, because of the natural levodopa action of the herb, it's very important to keep your practitioner informed about use of any Ayurvedic herbal approaches.

❖ HERBAL MEDICINE

When you pick up a bottle of echinacea off the supermarket shelf, or drink a ginger ale to settle your stomach, you're actually practicing herbal medicine. Going back to ancient times, there has always been an understanding of the power of plants and plant products as medicine. Many of today's most powerful and effective drugs actually come from plants and herbs or are synthetic versions of naturally occurring herbs. According to the World Health Organization (WHO), some four billion people, or 80 percent of the world's population, use some form of herbal medicine.

While always a mainstay in the East, and the basis for the remedies in both Traditional Chinese Medicine and Ayurveda, herbal medicine is becoming increasingly popular in the West, and herbal teas, supplements, extracts, and tinctures are all enjoying a resurgence.

In the United States, herbal medicine practitioners may be physicians, osteopaths, naturopaths, nutritionists, or more traditional "herbalists." But be particularly careful about reputation and credentials, and avoid so-called herbalists who are selling multilevel-marketed supplements and vitamins, as most are ill prepared to offer herbal or health advice.

When it comes to Parkinson's disease, herbal medicine is

frequently incorporated into overall nutritional advice as part of a program that focuses on detoxification, enhanced nutrition, and herb, vitamin, mineral, and amino acid supplementation. This comprehensive approach—as well as specific herbs that may be helpful to Parkinson's patients—is discussed in chapter 8.

❖ HOMEOPATHY

If you've seen a cold and flu remedy called Oscillococcinum on the drugstore shelf, you've seen contemporary homeopathic medicine in action. The current practice of homeopathy is based on two-hundred-year-old work of a German doctor, Samuel Hahnemann. Homeopathy's basic idea is that you can stimulate the body's own healing mechanisms to fight illness by administering a homeopathic remedy—a microscopic, extremely diluted amount of an herb, mineral, or other substance—that would cause similar symptoms in a healthy person. The theory is "like cures like," similar to the concept behind giving a vaccine that contains some elements of the disease the vaccination is meant to prevent.

Homeopathy was very popular in the United States in the late 1800s, and nearly 15 percent of all physicians at that time used homeopathy. The growth of the pharmaceutical industry put almost all homeopaths out of business until recently, when the popularity of homeopathy has returned. Currently, there are an estimated three thousand physicians and other health care personnel practicing homeopathy in the United States alone, and many more practitioners in Europe, Canada, and throughout the world.

Parkinson's disease patients should visit a licensed homeopath, who will conduct a lengthy interview about physical and psychological preferences and symptoms and then, based on an analysis of the responses, recommend a customized program of homeopathic remedies that can help with some symptoms of the condition.

Some of the homeopathic remedies a trained practitioner might recommend include the following:

- Anthimonium tartaricum—for trembling and tremor of head and hands
- Gelsemium—for trembling, droopy eyelids, staggering, weakness, and fatigue
- Mercurius corrosivus—for trembling hands and excessive salivation
- Agaricus—for stiff but trembling or twitching limbs, with itchy back and spine
- Hyoscyamus—for twitching, restlessness, and jealous/suspicious moods
- Rhus toxicodendron—for mild tremors and stiffness that lessens with movement

Finding a Homeopath

If you are looking for a homeopath, don't just accept someone's labeling himself or herself an expert. Be sure to find someone licensed to practice. There are a number of licenses that are awarded by accreditating organizations, including the following,

- D.Ht., Diplomate in Homeotherapeutics, which is given by the American Board of Homeotherapeutics to M.D.s and osteopaths who have practiced homeopathy for at least three years

- C.C.H., Certified in Classical Homeopathy, given by the Council for Homeopathic Certification
- D.H.A.N.P., Diplomate of the Homeopathic Academy of Naturopathic Physicians, given to naturopathic physicians who have completed at least 250 hours of homeopathic coursework and passed an exam

❖ RELAXATION, MEDITATION, AND STRESS REDUCTION

Sometimes, activities that reduce stress are referred to as "mind-body" medicine or "stress-reduction" therapies. But this category of activities generally encompass the full range of activities that seek to establish a link between conscious thought and the body, with the goal of affecting the body's processes or responses.

According to Harvard physician Herbert Benson, M.D., the nation's foremost mind-body expert, the objective of mind-body medicine is what he's termed the *relaxation response,* in which body functions become more balanced and actual physiological changes can be observed after the patient is brought to a relaxed state. In a radio interview with public-radio host Diane Rehm, Dr. Benson explained the relaxation response:

> We have found that when people regularly go into a quiet state, a large percentage of them feel the presence of a power, a force, an energy, God if you will, and they feel that presence is close to them, within them, [and] these people have fewer medical symptoms. Now, whether or not this is a physiological reaction independent of an external belief system, or whether or not

there is indeed something out there, we cannot answer,
but from the patient's point of view, they feel better.

While some experts point to the physical effects these activities can have, and others believe that the "spiritual" component is the key factor, there is some tendency to attribute the
effectiveness of these therapies to a placebo effect. That sort of
dismissal overlooks the real effectiveness of these techniques,
however, as there is a strong medical basis for mind-body therapy, and recent studies in psychoneuroimmunology show that
the mind can communicate with the nervous, immune, and
endocrine systems.

Research shows that mind-body techniques are particularly
useful in the stress-reduction areas, helping to reduce blood
pressure, pain, headaches, asthma, and other illnesses with a
strong stress component. Mind-body techniques are also empowering, involving you in your own health care as an active
participant.

There are so many types of mind-body therapy—everything from prayer to yoga to counseling to dance to breathing
exercises—that we can just touch upon a few. Some of the approaches that fall into this broad category include biofeedback,
guided imagery, hypnosis, transcendental meditation, psychotherapy, spiritual healing, music therapy, art therapy,
breathing exercises, and humor therapy, and other forms of relaxation all fall into this realm as well.

Ultimately, you'll need to more fully research those therapies that are most appealing to you, and where best to participate. But some of the mind-body aspects you may wish to
consider are summarized here.

Mind-Body Therapies and Options

By providing an outlet for stress and anxiety, psychotherapy or counseling can help to calm down your overall emotional state, allowing more energy for healing and fostering more positive thoughts and actions, which in turn speeds recovery.

Support groups provide an outlet for anxiety and stress, plus they have the added benefit of sometimes providing education and information that gives you a feeling of greater control. Studies have found that even people with fatal illnesses live far longer when part of a support group than those who did not participate in a support group. Keep in mind, however, that support groups come in all sizes and shapes. If you're interested in considering a support group, find one that will meet your needs. Be careful if you're young, newly diagnosed, or have mild Parkinson's, because a group of far older patients or those who have more serious and advanced symptoms may not be appropriate for you. Also, some groups are more like social groups than support groups for patients, so be sure to choose a group that fits your current needs.

Biofeedback is a treatment method that uses monitoring instruments that provide you with various physical information—such as pulse, body temperature, and other indicators of stress—which you normally don't monitor. By wearing the biofeedback monitor, you learn to adjust your thinking to then control bodily processes such as blood pressure, temperature, gastrointestinal functioning, and brain wave activity. These are normally not under your direct control physically.

Creative therapies, such as dance, music, or art therapy, use the creative arts—and in the case of dance therapy, the physical activity—to address health concerns. One study reported in 1998 found that a group of Parkinson's patients who received thirteen weekly two-hour sessions of music therapy—in which musical instruments were used to help elicit emotional and physical responses—had better motor function and often a decrease in hypokinesia. The study showed that music therapy had a beneficial effect on the emotional functions, activities of daily living, and quality of life of Parkinson's patients.

The famous physician Oliver Sacks, M.D., on whom the book and film *Awakenings* was based, has said this about music therapy:

> I regard music therapy as a tool of great power in many neurological disorders—Parkinson's and Alzheimer's—because of its unique capacity to organize or reorganize cerebral function when it has been damaged.

One benefit to the creative process, whether painting, drawing, singing, or playing music, is that it seems to tap into a different pathway in the brain for Parkinson's patients, many of whom find that symptoms lessen—or even disappear—when they are involved in a creative act. Colorado painter Mary Noone describes the experience:

> With Parkinson's, you're up one minute, then down the next. I go from points when I can't move, to points when I can enjoy a two-hour run in the mountains. But what happens with the painting, and this is purely from my own observation, is that when I paint, oftentimes my symptoms will cease. It's not like I can pick up a paintbrush and it will go away—if it did I would paint a whole lot more! But symptoms will often lessen and sometimes go away while I am painting.

One patient, Steve, has found that playing classical music on his piano both helps his fine motor coordination and calms his emotions. While playing, and for several hours afterward, his tremors actually go away.

Writing and journaling are other effective mind-body therapies. If you've ever written an e-mail, bulletin board post, journal or diary entry, or letter about something bothering you and felt better when you finished writing, you've experienced the positive power of writing. A 1999 study published in the *Journal of the American Medical Association* reported that some patients with chronic diseases had improvements in their health after writing about major life stresses.

Prayer and mental healing techniques usually describe an altered state of consciousness due to a spiritual experience, or the "flow of energy" or healing via another person's hands. Studies have shown these techniques can be effective, again particularly when it comes to stress and energy-related problems.

Meditation techniques are most common in Asia and are an integral part of Buddhism, Hinduism, many other Asian religions, and yoga, and have gained popularity in other countries in the past thirty years. Regular meditation or guided relaxation and imagery have notable effects on blood pressure, anxiety, chronic pain, body tension, and immune response and can clinically reduce cortisol levels, a measure of the body's stress level. Researchers have also shown, using magnetic resonance imaging (MRI), that meditation can activate certain structures in the brain that control the autonomic nervous system, a system that can become dysfunctional in some Parkinson's disease patients.

One patient, Dennis, 66, has had Parkinson's disease for eight years. Despite having to retire from a successful career as a car salesman, a divorce, and bankruptcy, Dennis has maintained a very positive state of mind. Says Dennis:

> I explained to my doctor that my frame of mind is so positive and balanced that I think I can deal with almost anything. I attribute this to meditation. I have been actively practicing meditation for the past eighteen years, long before I was diagnosed with Parkinson's. It is a part of me; I practice daily for an hour and intensely on Fridays and Saturdays for up to four hours and attend a meditation group and workshops. I was one of those triple-A personality types; people said I wouldn't live past 45. I would lose my temper all the time, overreact and try to control everything. Meditation changed all that. One of my friends recently said to me, "Your lows are my highs." I wish everyone could learn about the power of meditation and connecting to a higher power. It is life changing and helps you deal with anything, from bankruptcy to Parkinson's disease.

Guided imagery can be an effective technique for healing. You can use your own imagery or follow a book, audiotape or practitioner. If you are feeling stress, you might envision progressively relaxing each part of your body as you relax on a warm sunny beach, or you might envision the body's healing capabilities focusing on an organ or process that isn't working as optimally as possible.

To try a simple guided imagery exercise, close your eyes, take several deep, full abdominal breaths, and then focus on a particular symptom that is most troublesome to you right now. Allow an image to appear that represents your symptom. Don't judge the image that appears, just accept it and observe it. What feelings do you have about it? Tell the image how you feel about it, silently or out loud. Then visualize that the image is answering you, telling you why it's there, what it wants, what it's trying to tell you or do. Ask the image if it is willing to have your symptom abate. Then decide if you're willing to give the image what it wants. Continue the exchange until you feel that you've come to some sort of deal with the image.

One Parkinson's patient, Rita, uses relaxation and breathing exercises as her most important tactic.

The second most important thing is to have a place to "go" in your mind. It can be imaginary or an actual place. For me, being such a realist, I chose a real place in the front yard of our vacation home in Hawaii, under a palm tree on the ocean in the white sand. When I "go there," I can actually feel the warmth of the sun on my face, feel the trade winds, and hear the ocean washing in and out, in and out. Even though I don't spend any real-life time there now, I can still feel and see that place vividly in my mind. So what I do is close my eyes and concentrate on breathing from deep in my belly, visualize the breath traveling up through a channel next to my spine, up through my neck and then I put my tongue in the top of the mouth and softly blow the air out through my nose. The small noise of the air leaving my body sounds to me like the ocean lapping on the shore. I get a rhythm going, matching my breathing with the ocean coming and going, and then I start to feel the sun's warmth on my face. If you are totally concentrating on this, it is sort of a time-out for your brain from stress, etc., just like if your leg hurts and you prop it up for a time-out.

When I have a headache I visualize the pain "leaking" out when I exhale from wherever the center of the pain is, like through my eyelids. Just a few minutes of escape can turn the tide and get me on a new path for another chance to make it through whatever stress is on the menu at the time. I use this method to get to sleep at night.

◈ LAUGHTER THERAPY

Laughing is very important, as it can stimulate the release of natural endorphins, chemicals in the brain that can lessen pain and create a sense of well-being and a feeling of happiness. Prior studies on medical students showed that students who watched movies that were comedies had a boost in their immune system, with an increase in their white blood cell counts, compared to those who watched serious dramas. Some patients have found laughing to be very helpful. Some patients actually make an appointment to call a friend once a week and just laugh. One woman who did this regularly swore it made her feel so much better, her mood was happier, and that she even felt less stiff and slow on those days.

Another way to use laughter is to occasionally laugh at your symptoms or day-to-day dilemmas rather than become angry or frustrated. Elliot and his wife were able to do just that when dealing with the hallucinations Elliot was experiencing as a side effect of some of his medicines for Parkinson's disease. During a clinic visit, when asked if the hallucinations were bothersome to Elliot, he quickly said, "No," but his wife emphatically nodded yes. The doctor then asked what he saw when he hallucinated and he replied, "Four naked women in the shower." Everyone laughed!

❖ PHYSICAL THERAPY

Physical therapy focuses on prevention and treatment of a variety of conditions, with special emphasis on people who have lost movement or mobility as a result of illness or accident. Using exercise, movement, and even electrotherapy, physical therapists can help patients maintain as active a life as possible, with the greatest degree of physical independence. Overall, physical therapy can help with endurance, strength, and general fitness and energy level. It can also help improve mood, reducing anxiety and depression.

Physical therapy can have an important role in improving the treatment of Parkinson's disease and is particularly useful for stiffness, posture, rigidity, balance, and in helping people to get up from a chair or out of bed. Special physical therapy treatments can also be useful for those experiencing writhing movements and freezing—difficulty in initiating movement—which can result from the Parkinson's or the drug treatments.

According to Professor Rowena Plant of the Institute of Rehabilitation at the University of Northumbria in the United Kingdom:

> Physiotherapy [physical therapy] will never be a cure for Parkinson's disease, but it could have a profound role to play in managing the disease and minimizing its impact on everyday life. If physiotherapy is given to patients at an early stage, it can help to prepare the body for what will be a degenerative process. If you can get the body toned up, the disabling effects are likely to be less profound than they would otherwise be.

Experts looked at some of the best studies to date on physical therapy and Parkinson's disease and found that it does appear to offer some benefit to patients, particularly when one to three sessions are conducted each week. Some researchers, however, believe that, because physical therapy is costly and typically designed to continue only for several months (and after stopping, benefits seem to disappear), patients would be better served by a dedicated and ongoing long-term program of home exercise.

❖ MANUAL HEALING, BODYWORK, AND ENERGY WORK

Various types of manual healing, bodywork, and energy work can be of benefit to Parkinson's disease patients. There are so many different forms of massage and manual healing that it's hard to even list them all. Swedish massage, trigger-point massage (myotherapy, neuromuscular massage therapy), Rolfing, Trager, Alexander technique, Feldenkrais, myofascial release technique, and other realignment therapies concentrate on the soft tissue surrounding the bones. In bodywork and manual healing, hands, arms, elbows, and sometimes even feet are used to apply various types of touch or pressure to affect the muscles, bones, joints, circulation, and other body systems. Practitioners of reflexology and acupressure stimulate points so as to clear energy pathways that appear to be blocked. And there are many kinds of energy work, such as Reiki and Therapeutic Touch, in which the therapist is a conduit for healing energy that is directed to the patient through the therapist's hands, sometimes without actually touching the client.

But what they share in common is typically the use of touch for healing and well-being. If you've ever had a massage and enjoyed the relaxed, warm feeling it gave you for many hours afterward, you've appreciated the health benefits of manual healing and bodywork, which are some of the oldest methods of health care.

Massage therapy can be particularly beneficial for Parkinson's disease patients, due to its ability to relieve some joint and muscle stiffness, reduce stress, and increase the sense of well-being. The type of massage you choose truly depends on your own preferences—for example, some people prefer the more traditional Swedish massage, and others find shiatsu most relaxing and effective. The effects will vary due to your preferences and the particular skills and style of the practitioner, so you should try some different styles and practitioners until you find one that's the right fit. Be sure that your massage therapist is licensed and accredited. Deep-muscle massage is a form of bodywork that aims to stretch connective tissue around tight muscles to relieve cramping and improve mobility.

Some studies have shown that massage can naturally increase dopamine, the brain chemical that is depleted in Parkinson's disease. Maria Hernandez-Reif, Ph.D., of the University of Miami Touch Research Institute, in an interview with *Ivanhoe Newswire,* said that simple massage could help Parkinson's disease. Says Dr. Hernandez-Reif, "We're finding that it helps the Parkinson's patients sleep better, and it improves their daily living activity."

Acupressure, or pressure-point massage, can help some Parkinson's patients with symptoms such as nausea, excessive salivation, anxiety, and muscle rigidity and pain. Acupressure can also help improve energy and relieve fatigue.

Craniosacral massage is a type of massage that focuses on light touch and acupressure to the head. The theory behind it is that it releases tension and restores energy balance. One patient, Louise, 78, has had Parkinson's disease for five years. She is on very low doses of Sinemet three times a day as her only medication for Parkinson's disease, and swears by this form of massage as part of her treatment.

> I have been getting craniosacral massage therapy almost every week for the last two years. I know it is making my body healthier and helping the Parkinson's disease. I am not as stiff or slow as I was before I started craniosacral massage, and I do not need or want more medicine for Parkinson's disease.

Osteopathic manipulation works with the musculoskeletal system as a way to treat illness, which, in osteopathic theory, can result from imbalances and misalignment in the body's structure. In osteopathic manipulation, the physician manually applies force to various parts of the body as a way to improve function, realign and balance the musculoskeletal system, and restore balance to various body systems. It's typically helpful for muscular and skeletal pain and in some cases is used to help deal with symptoms, or even underlying causes, of certain conditions. Some M.D. practitioners have also been trained in osteopathic manipulation and can provide this sort of therapy. There is clear research supporting the use of osteopathic manipulation and techniques for musculoskeletal and nonmusculoskeletal problems.

Some Parkinson's patients have found the Feldenkrais method of bodywork particularly helpful. Feldenkrais involves exercises, usually performed with a practitioner, that help to improve the body's autonomic motor responses—which can be adversely affected by Parkinson's disease.

There are many forms of energy work, in which practitioners transfer "healing energy" to recipients, but one of the most popular and effective appears to Reiki, pronounced "ray-key." Reiki teacher, practitioner, and holistic healer Phylameana lila Desy has described Reiki as a vibrational healing modality that consists of an enormous amount of what she terms "love energy." In Reiki some practitioners touch recipients, while others just pass hands over the body. But the central tenet behind Reiki is that the practitioner is tapping into a universal "energy force" and then passing that energy on to the recipient, who will receive it where it is most needed—mind or body. Says Desy:

> I teach my students that Reiki is a "smart energy" because it works at the level of acceptance by each individual client. Reiki will never overwhelm someone who is not accustomed to feeling energy, as it will enter the body slowly. For someone more open to the energy, it will flow more quickly, but only at the level that is needed. Reiki is a balancing remedy. It will flow directly to whatever is in imbalance and nudge it back into a more balanced state. Visualize the swing of a pendulum and perhaps you will understand what I am trying to convey. Depending on how out of balance something is, Reiki (the swing of the pendulum) will adjust itself accordingly. Naturally someone with a chronic problem did not get this condition overnight, so they would be in error to expect Reiki to bring about 100 percent alignment of body imbalances following a single session. Reiki will address physical imbalances first before addressing the emotional, mental, and spiritual problems. For this reason alone, I think the benefits someone with a chronic illness could ex-

perience from consistent Reiki treatments are the receiving of relief from the physical and emotional suffering.

❖ EXERCISE

Exercise is an essential complementary therapy for most Parkinson's patients. Because movements are affected in Parkinson's disease, exercise can be an important part of treatment. While it won't stop the progress of Parkinson's disease, it may improve muscle and joint strength, maximize one's physical ability and prevent further degeneration and disability due to disuse or injury.

Some doctors recommend muscle-strengthening exercises to help Parkinson's disease patients tone muscles and to encourage greater mobility and range of motion in underused and rigid muscles. Exercise can also improve balance, help with walking problems, and even improve speaking and swallowing. Exercise also elevates mood and can help relieve depression and foster feelings of general well-being.

The form of exercise you choose depends on your own preferences and your mobility, but ideally you should pick an exercise that you can do regularly throughout the year and that gets your muscles moving and increases heart rate. Walking, jogging, stretching, swimming, and other activities can help Parkinson's patients. Be sure to consult your doctor before starting any exercise program, however, and don't exercise when you feel tired.

One patient, Chris, has incorporated exercise into the overall Parkinson's disease treatment program. Says Chris:

I try to exercise daily. I alternate aerobic exercise on a stationary bike three days a week with yoga one day a week, t'ai chi one day a week, and do fifteen minutes of muscle stretches a day. These exercises help my muscle tone, improve my strength, and increase my energy level and state of mind. It gives me a sense of being able to impact my health by keeping my body as healthy as I can and not just relying on a pill to do that.

Mary Noone, a 45-year-old artist in a small town in the Colorado mountains, believes that exercise and physical activity are critical to her health and ability to function. She takes time for hiking and running in the mountains several times a week and says that except for her Parkinson's disease, she's in the best shape of her life.

I just had a checkup a few weeks ago, and the doctor gave me an absolute clean bill of health. My blood pressure, cholesterol—they're all perfect. I'm five foot nine and am now skinnier than I've ever been, mainly because I'm moving all the time. My muscles are very defined. I've gotten much more physical activity since having the Parkinson's.

One group of researchers found that patients with stages I through III Parkinson's disease who participated in a ten-week strength-training program and balance exercises focusing on the lower limbs showed significantly improved balance, as well as some improvement in knee flexibility and strength. A control group that did not perform exercise had no improvement in balance and a significant reduction in strength.

The National Parkinson Foundation publishes a helpful 58-page manual, *Parkinson's Disease: Fitness Counts,* that features exercises Parkinson's patients can do on their own at home. Another good resource is the book *Parkinson's Disease and the Art of Moving,* from John Argue, which provides a comprehensive exercise program designed specifically for Parkinson's disease patients. And some Parkinson's disease patients who are in more advanced stages of the disease swear by a program developed by Jodi Stolove, called "Chair Dancing," which consists of seated aerobic exercise that improves muscle tone, flexibility, and cardiovascular endurance. Information about all these materials is featured in Appendix A.

◆ YOGA AND T'AI CHI

Some of the gentle stretching and balance-oriented exercises such as yoga and t'ai chi are ideal for Parkinson's patients because they involve slow, deliberate movements. They are not competitive, and emphasize performing physical movements slowly, deliberately, with mindfulness and awareness. As exercises that have mind-body aspects, they also help with mood and depression.

When most people think of yoga, they assume it means stretching or sitting around in a cross-legged lotus position. Yoga is actually an ancient science that focuses on finding a balance and harmony among the whole body, mind, and spirit and with the universe. Yoga combines physical exercises (known as *asanas*), breathing exercises (*pranayama*), and meditation techniques to help achieve that union and balance.

Some of the many health benefits of yoga have been conventionally tested and proven and are even discussed in the Western medical journals. For example, certain forms of yoga have been found to have a strong antidepressant effect. Yoga has also been found to improve lung function and breathing. Yoga is also considered an effective treatment for carpal tunnel syndrome. These are just a few of the many practical applications even mainstream medicine has found for yoga.

Dina, a caregiver for her mother, who has Parkinson's disease, has this to say about yoga:

I started taking my mom to the yoga classes and I can honestly say it has improved her muscle stiffness and flexibility. Also, she gets a real benefit from socializing with other Parkinson's disease patients that go to the class. She has made some good friends there. She also seems more alert in the afternoon after going to class.

Wanda Barnes, a registered nurse and certified Kripalu yoga instructor, conducts yoga classes in the Jacksonville, Florida, area, including a class specially designed for Parkinson's disease patients. Wanda believes that yoga can be a wonderful addition to a Parkinson's disease patient's regular program of exercise.

Most Parkinson's patients are capable of enjoying a gentle, beginner yoga class, but may require some adaptation of modification to accommodate their limitations. What I teach is very basic, modified yoga. Most of it is done sitting in a chair, rather than a mat. We do some things on the mat, but it's limited. We've learned to modify, so we do a lot of the class sitting in the chair and standing, until the final part of class, which is conducted in relaxation pose, lying on mat.

Wanda has seen some positive benefits for her students.

One man said something that really struck me—he said, "We come, we enjoy it, but it really changes my attitude. Makes it easier to accept what your life situation is." Another lady had a really profound experience. She started the class able to sleep only two hours a night, maximum. Just a few weeks into the class, she reported that she was able to relax so deeply that she was sleeping through the night for the first time in a long time. And one of our patients, who concentrated on deep breathing, conscious relaxation, and guided imagery, has learned to have greater control over his tremors, to let them subside and sometimes even stop them.

In addition to these success stories, Wanda finds that yoga helps her students in other ways.

It helps you be more conscious of how you move, have more awareness of where you have stress, where you have areas that are tense, where you have pain, and that you have the ability to work with that and release some of it, through stretching and relaxing.

Wanda also encourages caregivers, friends, and other support people to consider attending classes with the Parkinson's patients, as part of their own self-care routine.

There are a variety of styles and classes of yoga, so choosing the one that is right for you may require a bit of research. Yoga classes at different levels are widely available at yoga centers, health clubs, community centers, rehabilitation centers, and many other locations. For a Parkinson's patient considering yoga, Wanda recommends talking to the person actually teaching the class—not a receptionist—to discuss what style they teach. Ask the teacher how they modify the class for people who can't do everything sitting on a mat.

Do they have chairs available, and will they incorporate them into the class for those who have difficulty moving from standing to sitting on the mat frequently? Ask how challenging the class would be for someone who doesn't have the flexibility of the joints and who maybe can't perform all the exercises. Maybe even go to a class, find out how long it is, and watch and see what kinds of things they are doing before you start.

As with any exercise, the more you can practice outside the class, the more benefit you will enjoy. Wanda even believes that future studies will show that regular practice of yoga for Parkinson's patients not only reduces pain and increases flexibility, but may even slow down the progression of rigidity and stiffness.

T'ai chi, also known as t'ai chi ch'uan, is a form of exercise that originated in China. T'ai chi coordinates movements of the body with the mind and breathing and emphasizes flexibility, balance, and serenity of both mind and body. In one study, it was found that people who practiced t'ai chi had improved balance, flexibility, and cardiovascular fitness when compared to sedentary Parkinson's patients. Other studies have shown that t'ai chi can improve balance in older practitioners. A 1997 study at Atlanta's Emory University found that a fifteen-week modified t'ai chi program significantly reduced falls in a group of older seniors.

Patients who practice t'ai chi on a regular basis report that they are sleeping better, have improved energy levels, and have an improved sense of balance. Some patients have enjoyed a reduction in their rate of falling or stumbling, and one patient stopped using her cane and walker after three months of practicing t'ai chi. Results from a single-blinded study of t'ai chi and Parkinson's disease reported that patients who over a three-month period attended t'ai chi classes two times a week, and practiced on their own three additional days per week, were eighteen times less likely to fall, compared to other patients who didn't practice t'ai chi.

One Parkinson's patient, Tom, had a positive experience with t'ai chi.

My biggest fear is falling. I've learned that the floor is very hard. The part of not being able to control my fall is my big problem. Once I start to go forward, I can't do anything to stop it. When I started going to t'ai chi class, it was wonderful. I learned how to be more aware of my balance and how to move more efficiently to lessen the risk of falling. It took about two months of classes before I really started to notice a difference. I'm not falling as much . . . I used to fall three to four times a week and now I mostly stumble without falling at all or at most fall once a month. T'ai chi has made the difference.

Sylvia attended t'ai chi regularly for one year and says it was probably a lifesaver for her.

I have several dogs. One day, my one-hundred-pound lab took out after my cat. I set out after the dog, grabbed her by the collar, and somehow managed to get my hand stuck in her collar. I have never moved so fast in my life—the dog just kept going. All I could think about was falling and breaking every bone in my body. In the process of my adventure, I kept saying, "T'ai chi, balance," over and over again, "Balance, t'ai chi." I finally worked my hand out of the collar and was still running, then started to slow down and managed to be all together without having fallen. I said, "Thank you, God, thank you, t'ai chi." A year ago I didn't know what t'ai chi was; I learned about it from a holistic symposium on Parkinson's. I am very grateful for the opportunity to practice t'ai chi.

❖ NATUROPATHY

Naturopathy seeks to identify and treat root causes of illness or the disease process instead of symptoms. Naturopaths may recommend or may themselves practice acupuncture, homeopathy, herbal medicine, dietary and nutritional medicine, manipulation or massage, and other techniques. Naturopathic philosophy aims for a balance of physical, emotional, mental, and spiritual aspects, highlighting the body's innate ability to heal itself. Naturopathic doctors frequently act as "primary care providers" for many complementary and alternative therapies and are often well connected to a network of alternative providers.

Since naturopathic medicine draws on many different disciplines, there are certainly arguments to be made for its effectiveness. But since there are no specific "naturopathic" remedies or treatments, it really is up to the individual practitioner to achieve results, so getting recommendations from other practitioners or patients is particularly important here.

It's estimated that there are more than one thousand naturopathic doctors in practice in the United States. If you are looking for a reputable naturopath, it's best to consult with someone who has an "N.D." certification and is a licensed Doctor of Naturopathic Medicine. The Council on Naturopathic Medical Education grants this designation after completion of a four-year program at one of the several accredited naturopathic colleges in the United States.

❖ OPENING YOUR MIND

The most important thing of all is to open your mind to the possibility of one or more of the above therapies as a means of healing and promoting physical, emotional, and spiritual health. You will need to explore various therapies to find what works for you and what does not. Trust your instincts—practice what feels right and discard what does not.

Chapter 8

Dietary, Nutritional, Vitamin, Enzyme, and Hormone Therapies

The human body has been designed to resist an infinite number of changes and attacks brought about by its environment. The secret of good health lies in successful adjustment to changing stresses on the body.

—Harry J. Johnson

Practitioners of complementary and alternative medicine view Parkinson's disease as a condition of toxic overloads, inflammation, insufficient nutrition to the brain, and various nutritional deficiencies. How these various triggers are assessed and treated will differ, depending on whether you see an Ayurvedic practitioner, who might recommend Ayurvedic remedies that contain various herbs and nutrients, or a nutritionist, who might develop a plan for diet and supplements to address your condition, or a functional medicine expert, who might test for various deficiencies, pathogens, and toxins before developing a detoxification/nutrition/treatment plan, including diet, exercise, stress reduction, hormones, herbs, and vitamin and mineral supplements.

There is no standard recommendation for Parkinson's patients, because a diet-and-supplements plan should always be customized for your own condition. There's a temptation to head down to the drugstore or health food store to stock up on various supplements you hear about, but self-treatment is not recommended for Parkinson's disease patients. You'll have better, safer results by consulting with a holistic physician, nutritionist, herbalist, or other expert in conjuction with your regular doctor, to develop a customized plan. Professionally developed recommendations can help you maximize and enhance your wellness, avoid any interactions between supplements and other drugs you are taking, and prevent any worsening of your condition.

❖ PATHWAYS TO PARKINSON'S

In order to understand how diet, nutrition, and lifestyle changes may help Parkinson's patients, it is essential to explore some of the physiological and biochemical changes that may be part of the Parkinson's disease process—changes that may be responsive to natural or holistic approaches.

Dr. Catherine Willner is an innovative physician who has studied the degenerative processes that can lead to nervous system diseases such as Parkinson's. Dr. Willner believes that there are four possible pathways that are responsible, including chronic inflammation, mitochondrial dysfunction, endocrine imbalances, and hypomethylation.

Chronic Inflammation

Inflammation is thought to increase the risk of blood clots in the brain, increase the risk of brain damage, and release pro-inflammatory chemicals throughout the body. Inflammation in the brain and other parts of the body may increase the risk of Parkinson's or trigger the condition in susceptible individuals. Some groups taking anti-inflammatory drugs for other conditions have actually shown a substantial reduction in the risk of Parkinson's disease and other neurodegenerative diseases. Because of the neurological risk of inflammation, combined with the fact that inflammation reduces the immune system's ability to repair damaged cells, reducing inflammation is an important part of possibly avoiding or slowing down or improving Parkinson's disease. Chronic inflammation is dealt with by identifying and dealing with various sources of inflammation—including food allergens, pathogens, and infectious organisms—and introducing anti-inflammatory foods, supplements, and ways of eating, such as the low-glycemic diet.

Mitochondrial Dysfunction

The brain has a high requirement for energy and therefore has a higher density of mitochondria, the cell's energy producers, than other parts of the body. According to Barbara Maddoux, a Doctor of Oriental Medicine and an expert on nutrition and holistic therapies for Parkinson's patients, mitochondria are the energy factories of the cell and are abundant in the brain. The brain uses 20 percent of the total oxygen consumed by the body, which is quite a high percentage, when considering that the brain comprises only 2 percent of body weight. With so much oxygen consumption, more free radicals are produced in the brain cells. Says Dr. Maddoux:

The brain cells are deficient in the enzyme systems that can neutralize these free radicals. And, when you consider the additional burden of toxic exposure, household chemicals, lawn and garden sprays, and pesticides and toxins on food and in commercially raised meat and dairy, the already overburdened mitochondria soon grind to a painfully slow pace in their ability to produce energy, protect against free radical damage, and promote optimum health.

Supporting healthy mitochondrial energy production is therefore an important part of a holistic protocol for Parkinson's disease.

Supporting mitochondrial function, according to Dr. Maddoux, relies on first preventing, or at least diminishing, further toxic exposures. Second, antioxidants are needed to help protect the body and brain cells from free-radical damage.

Endocrine Imbalance

Dr. Willner and other experts believe that the body's difficulty adapting to stress can in some people result in chronically elevated glucocorticoids—i.e., cortisol—which can be detrimental to the brain and trigger neurological decline and imflammatory processes. Typically, these endocrine imbalances are usually evident in prediabetic-type conditions such as hyerglycemia and hypoglycemia. Balancing the endocrine system is therefore another important part of a holistic program for Parkinson's disease. Solutions for endocrine imbalance include the addition of exercise, which can help with blood sugar, a low-glycemic diet, maximizing digestion, and use of appropriate supplements to aid in balancing blood sugar.

Hypomethylation

Some experts believe that the brain depends on a steady supply of nutrients, in particular, folic acid and vitamins B_{12} and B_6. In the brain, folate (folic acid) goes through a conversion process in which it combines with homocysteine and utilizes vitamin B_{12} to produce the precursor to S-adenosylmethionine (SAMe), which is necessary for proper brain and nervous system functioning. The overall process is known as methylation. When there are insufficient levels of the B vitamins, the entire process is inhibited, which is known as hypomethylation, and it's theorized that hypomethylation can lead to a variety of problems with neurological function.

Hypomethylation is considered a marker for aging, and is also commonly seen with elevated homocysteine levels, which is a risk for heart disease. Addressing hypomethylation is, according to Dr. Willner, important to a Parkinson's disease wellness program. Dr. Willner's recommendation for hypomethylation is daily intake of a combination of supplements at the same time, including 650 micrograms of folic acid, 400 micrograms of vitamin B_{12}, and 10 milligrams of vitamin B_6.

❖ KEY RECOMMENDATIONS

Based on Dr. Willner's theories, there are a variety of nutritional suggestions that can be of help to Parkinson's patients. Again, optimally, patients should consult with a holistic or nutritional expert for a customized evaluation and program, but some of these guidelines are commonsense general guidelines that can aid in good health for most Parkinson's patients.

General Dietary Recommendations

Generally, Parkinson's disease patients should eat a well-balanced diet, high in fruits and vegetables and lower in protein. People with Parkinson's disease can benefit by avoiding or minimizing the following:

- Alcohol
- Coffee
- Caffeinated tea
- Sugar and sweetened foods
- Aspartame and other artificial sweeteners
- Processed foods with added chemicals
- Margarine, fats, fried foods, polyunsaturated oils
- Chlorinated and fluoridated water
- Some patients are particularly sensitive to very spicy hot foods, and have reported that they experience uncontrollable physical movement after eating them, so some patients will need to avoid these foods.

It's also critical to avoid tobacco and any unnecessary drugs.

Reduce Toxic Exposures, Choose Organic and Pesticide-Free Foods

A Parkinson's patient whose job or geographic location causes frequent exposure to pesticides or chemicals should consider finding a new job or location that minimizes exposure to environmental and chemical toxins. Another important part of limiting exposures is to drink only purified, filtered water—not tap water. It's essential to drink at least six to eight 8-ounce glasses of pure water daily, to help maintain proper water balance, enhance digestion, prevent constipation, and flush out toxins from the body. Parkinson's disease patients should particularly avoid drinking well water, as there is some linkage between a history of drinking well water and increased risk of Parkinson's disease. And finally, people with Parkinson's disease should, as often as possible, choose organic, unsprayed fruits and vegetables, as well as organic grains, dairy products, and meats. This minimizes ongoing exposure to residues from pesticides, as well as excess hormones and antibiotics.

Identify and Treat Food Sensitivities and Allergies

One important way to reduce chronic inflammation is to determine whether you have food allergies or sensitivities. Among foods, the most common allergens are

- Wheat and wheat gluten products,
- Dairy foods,
- Corn,
- Soy,
- Fish (especially shellfish),
- Nuts, and
- Fruits.

Allergies to particular foods can irritate and inflame the gastrointestinal system, creating an easy pathway for large food particles or pathogens to pass through the intestines, a condition frequently referred to as "leaky gut syndrome." Overexposure to insufficiently digested foods and inability to fight off the pathogens then sets up further allergies and inflammatory reactions. One way to identify food allergies is to follow an elimination diet, in which you remove an item completely from your diet for two weeks. Then you eat a large amount of the food you're testing, to see if you have any noticeable reaction over the subsequent seventy-two hours. Typical allergic reactions include diarrhea, nausea, gas, headache, rashes, skin eruptions, itching, fatigue, irritability, and other strong reactions or symptoms.

More-formalized allergy tests are also available from physicians and allergists, including skin tests and food allergy blood tests.

Eliminate Pathogens and Infection

It's not uncommon that the body is infected by bacteria, yeast, parasites, or other pathogens that may not be obvious, yet cause inflammation throughout the body. One useful process to consider is, under the guidance of an experienced practitioner, having selected testing to look for infectious organisms and pathogens. Some of the "stealth" infections that might be causing chronic inflammation include

- *Helicobacter pylori (H. pylori)*—the bacteria that causes ulcers;
- Gastrointestinal infections with bacteria such as *Yersinia enterocolitica* or *giardia*;
- *Candida albicans*—yeast overgrowth; and
- *Mycoplasma*—which can cause autoimmune symptoms and rheumatoid arthritis.

This sort of testing usually requires that you consult with a practitioner who specializes in what's known as "functional medicine." Functional-medicine practitioners may be M.D.s, nutritionists, naturopaths, or other types of holistic practitioners, but their emphasis is on uncovering the causes of symptoms, using laboratory assessment, with the goal of early intervention and treatment to improve health. Nutritional status, metabolism, and the presence of bacteria and pathogens are all evaluated, and deficiencies and imbalances are identified so that they can be corrected.

Consider a Low-Glycemic Diet

Doctor of Oriental Medicine Barbara Maddoux believes that reducing inflammation and balancing the endocrine system both require a diet that optimally balances blood sugar. Dr. Maddoux, like many innovative holistic practitioners, believes that sugar in the diet is an immune irritant and trigger for inflammation. To that end, Dr. Maddoux recommends that Parkinson's patients focus on eating smaller meals, more frequently, with a balance in protein, carbohydrate, and fat to minimize fluctuations in blood sugar. This approach is what's known as a low-glycemic diet. The glycemic index (GI) assigns a number to carbohydrate-based foods, based on how they affect your blood sugar. Foods with a lower GI cause only a slight increase in blood sugar, medium-range GI causes a higher increase in blood sugar, and high-glycemic foods cause blood sugar to rise significantly. A low-GI diet has been shown to help control blood sugar. When it comes to GI ratings, particularly with grains, it's a safe bet to look for foods with a high-fiber content. Higher-fiber breads, for example, have a lower GI than lower-fiber breads. Refined carbohydrates, such as white bread or pastas, tend to have a higher glycemic index but lower fiber. For a healthy approach to a low-glycemic diet, see the book *The Glucose Revolution: The Authoritative Guide to the Glycemic Index—The Groundbreaking Medical Discovery,* by Thomas M. S. Wolever, M.D., Ph.D., Jennie Brand-Miller,

Ph.D. (editor), Kaye Foster-Powell, and Stephen Colagiuri, M.D.; and Sandra Woodruff's *The Good Carb Cookbook: Secrets of Eating Low on the Glycemic Index*. Both of these books provide guidance on following a low-glycemic diet.

Maximize Your Digestion

Ensuring proper digestion is an important part of balancing the endocrine system and reducing inflammation. Large, undigested food particles carry a higher risk of setting off allergic responses, so it's important not only to chew food completely, but to consider supplementation with digestive enzymes that help to break down protein. Such a supplement program should include pepsin, betaine hydrochloride, and bromelain.

Another important thing to do to aid digestion is to take a probiotic supplement. Probiotics are supplements that contain live bacteria—the "good" bacteria found in fermented foods such as miso and dairy products such as yogurt and some cheeses—which the intestinal system normally contains in sufficient quantities. One of the more well-known bacteria in this category is acidophilus, the live cultures found in yogurt. Probiotics boost the activity of various disease-killing immune system cells and balance the intestinal bacteria environment to help minimize inflammation. Probiotics are typically available as a capsule supplement or as a powder that you can add to foods and drinks, and can be purchased at vitamin and health food stores and some pharmacies.

Eat "Good Fats" and Avoid "Bad Fats"

Many nutritional experts believe that the type of fat you eat has more of an impact on your overall health than the total fat intake. Saturated fats—found in meats, butter, and tropical oils—can contribute to inflammation and increased cholesterol, while the protective fats—such as those found in olive oil, avocados, fish, and nuts—can help protect against heart disease and reduce inflammation. From a dietary standpoint, you should avoid trans-monounsaturated fatty acids and hydrogenated fats. These are the fats found in shortening, margarine, snacks such as crackers and cookies, and in the oils used by fast-food restaurants. If the label says "partially hydrogenated," that's also a sign that it contains a trans-fatty acid.

Good fats primarily include the omega-3 fatty acids, such as those found in certain fish, which are shown to reduce inflammation. The fish-oil–based supplements EPA and DHA are a good source, but the optimal sources of these fats are oily fish such as salmon, tuna, herring, sardines, mackerel, and anchovies. Some experts say you need to be careful about the type of fish you eat, however. Some practitioners advise against eating certain fish which have been identified by the U.S. Environmental Protection Agency as being high in toxins. These fish include swordfish, shark, and mackerel. Other practitioners are more conservative and claim that only fish lowest in toxins should be eaten. These include summer flounder, wild Pacific salmon, croaker, sardines, haddock, and tilapia. Try to choose ocean fish over fish raised in fish farms, as farm-raised fish have far less omega 3s.

Eat More Fiber

Constipation is common in Parkinson's disease, so fiber in the diet is particularly important. The term *dietary fiber* refers to plant materials that are not easily digested. Fiber helps to normalize bowel function and can help prevent toxins from spending too much time in the intestines. Toxins that remain in the intestines for too long can potentially be absorbed into the bloodstream. Fiber also helps to limit the spike in blood sugar that typically occurs after eating, and can balance blood sugar. Most of us eat only 15 grams of fiber a day, but almost everyone should be eating 25 to 30 grams per day, perhaps even more for Parkinson's disease patients. To add fiber, choose higher-fiber versions of foods over lower-fiber versions—for example, the actual fruits versus juices, prunes, and other dried fruits; whole grains over refined grains; and higher-fiber fruits and vegetables such as berries and sweet potatoes. If you still can't get enough fiber into your diet, consider a fiber supplement. When you switch to a high-fiber diet or supplements, add them to your diet slowly over time, in order to minimize temporary side effects, which could include gas, cramps, and diarrhea.

 ## SPECIAL DIETARY SITUATIONS

Weight Loss

Weight loss can be a concern for some patients with Parkinson's disease. In some patients, this is due to excessive tremor or dyskinesia, which increases metabolism and burns more calories. Even in patients without these symptoms, weight loss often occurs despite an adequate diet. A dietitian or nutritionist can help modify the diet and recommend changes that will slow weight loss or help regain needed weight.

Dietary Protein and Wearing Off

As many as half of all Parkinson's disease patients find that after several years on carbidopa/levodopa, the effectiveness of their drug treatment wears off before they are scheduled to take their next dose. The result is the on-off cycling, in which patients have good times during the day—periods during which their drugs are working—followed by more symptomatic periods after the drug wears off and before they can take their next dose.

It's important to note that very large meals or meals high in fat may slow down the digestive system and therefore slow down or interfere with the absorption of the carbidopa/levodopa. So Parkinson's patients should eat smaller, more frequent meals and avoid high-fat foods and meals.

Another important aspect that affects the wearing off is the amount of protein eaten. After eating protein, it's broken down to amino acids, which then need to be digested. Levodopa is also an amino acid. When higher amounts of protein are eaten, the digestion of the protein's amino acids can get in the way of proper absorption of the levodopa, with negative consequences. Excessive protein can cause the carbidopa/levodopa to take longer to work, be less effective, and it may cause the carbidopa/levodopa to wear off more quickly. At the same time, while protein has the ability to interfere with response to levodopa, carbohydrates have been found to enhance absorption into the brain, given their ability to remove competing amino acids.

Protein cannot be removed from the diet entirely, as it's needed for proper nutrition. To that end, there are two key ways to get sufficient protein, while minimizing wearing-off responses. One is to eat carbohydrate meals during the day and restrict protein to little or none during the day, and consume the remaining daily intake of protein during the evening meal, when the symptomatic effects of the interaction with the carbidopa/levodopa drugs may be less inconvenient. This approach can be a help to some patients who are particularly sensitive to protein. Some patients do not prefer this approach, however, as they experience substantially reduced mobility in the evening.

Another option is what's known as the "7:1 plan." This involves eating meals that consist of a ratio of seven parts carbohydrate to one part protein. This plan may be easier for some patients, as it allows for small amounts of protein throughout the day, and with each meal.

The 7:1 plan requires that you focus primarily on a high-carbohydrate diet, with fruits, vegetables, and grains as the primary components of each meal and with just a small amount of protein—i.e., meat, poultry, eggs, fish, or dairy products—as a minor component.

An excellent resource to help you in determining an optimal diet to deal with wearing off is a book, *Eat Well, Stay Well with Parkinson's Disease,* by Kathrynne Holden, M.S., R.D. Once you've read this book and looked at the options, determining the optimal menu plan is something you should discuss with your physician and, ideally, with a registered dietitian or nutritionist who can help you plan and refine your optimal diet and meal plans. In particular, you need to discuss the 7:1 plan in advance, as some conditions—including diabetes and high triglycerides—may preclude following this plan or may require it to be modified.

❖ NUTRITIONAL AND HERBAL SUPPLEMENTS FOR PARKINSON'S DISEASE

There are a variety of supplements that may be a help to Parkinson's patients in terms of overall wellness, immune response, and brain and neurological health, and also for specific

Parkinson's disease or drug-related symptoms. In addition, key supplements address the major pathways mentioned earlier, including inflammation, mitochondrial dysfunction, endocrine imbalance, hypomethylation, and the underlying need for high levels of antioxidants.

Here is an overview of some of the key supplements that are frequently recommended for Parkinson's disease patients.

Vitamins

MULTIVITAMINS

A high-potency multivitamin and mineral supplement is something that most patients can take daily, to help ensure that basic minimum requirements of essential nutrients are met. It's best to take a vitamin in a form that is easily digested, such as a soft gel-cap.

VITAMIN D

Some practitioners feel that Parkinson's disease patients can benefit from vitamin D supplementation, particularly to help ward off the risk of osteoporosis. A usual dosage recommendation for vitamin D is 400 international units (IU) daily.

B-COMPLEX VITAMINS

The B vitamins are important to brain and nerve health. Parkinson's disease patients may want to take a multivitamin B-complex supplement daily. The debate about the benefits and risks of B_6 (pyridoxine) for use in Parkinson's disease is discussed in more detail later in this chapter. Current opinion is that up to 100 milligrams daily of B_6 is safe to take.

Vitamins C and E

Vitamins C and E are powerful antioxidants that fight free radicals. One study found that the newly diagnosed patients might be able to delay the start of carbidopa/levodopa treatment when they take high daily doses of the antioxidant combination of vitamins C and E. This sort of megavitamin therapy should be done only with an expert practitioner's guidance. Outside of megavitamin therapy, these supplements can individually be helpful for Parkinson's patients. Vitamin C can also help counteract the side effects—particularly nausea—of carbidopa/levodopa in some patients, and some practitioners claim that it helps reduce the frequency of on-off attacks. Experts recommend starting with 1,000 milligrams of vitamin C with bioflavonoids three times a day, for a month. At that point, slowly increase intake to the highest level that can be tolerated, up to 2,000 milligrams (2 grams). With vitamin E, a product containing mixed tocopherols should be used, and a recommended dose is 200 IU daily, gradually increasing to 400 IU in the morning and 400 IU in the evening.

Note: Parkinson's disease patients who have high blood pressure or who are on an anticoagulant (blood thinner) such as Coumadin (Warfarin) should not take vitamin E supplements without your physician's approval.

Minerals

Calcium and Magnesium

Calcium and magnesium are important for a healthy nervous system and can help with muscle cramps and rigidity. At minimum, 1,000 milligrams of calcium and 500 milligrams of magnesium a day are important. Some practitioners recommend as much as 800 to 1,200 milligrams of magnesium each day. Magnesium should be chelated or taken as magnesium chloride.

ZINC AND COPPER

People with Parkinson's disease are more likely to have imbalances in levels of both zinc and copper. Chronically low or high levels of these two minerals may make the brain more at risk of damage from free radicals and therefore cause an elevated risk of developing Parkinson's disease. A practitioner should advise regarding customized recommendations on these minerals, but minimum daily requirements are 15 milligrams a day for zinc and 1.5 to 3.0 milligrams a day for copper.

SELENIUM

Selenium is an antioxidant that can help increase circulation and tissue oxygenation, which helps to protect nerve cells from damage. Some experts suggest 200 micrograms (note *micrograms,* not milligrams) of selenium daily.

Digestive Help

PROBIOTICS

The "good" or friendly bacteria you find in yogurt and other foods can help ensure a healthy gastrointestinal tract, maximize the ability to properly absorb nutrients, help heal "leaky gut" syndrome, and ward off constipation. Sold as "Probiotics" supplements—or sometimes referred to by their names, acidophilus and bifidus bacteria—the supplements are available in capsules or powder form. Follow the label or your practitioner's instructions on when and how much to take.

DIGESTIVE ENZYMES

People with Parkinson's disease may not be utilizing nutrients effectively, due to incomplete digestion. Digestive enzyme supplements can help ensure complete digestion and assimilation of the nutrients in foods. A combination digestive enzyme supplement can be taken with meals as directed.

Other Supplements

GAMMA-AMINO BUTYRIC ACID (GABA)

Gamma-amino butyric acid (GABA) is an amino acid that functions as a neurotransmitter. GABA is a brain nutrient and can help strengthen the nervous system. Some practitioners recommend as much as 500 milligrams up to three times daily for three-month-long periods.

ALPHA-LIPOIC ACID (ALA)

Alpha-lipoic acid is an antioxidant supplement that can help other antioxidants function more effectively in the body. According to Dr. Barbara Maddoux, alpha-lipoic acid crosses the blood-brain barrier and is fat- and water-soluble. Not only is it an antioxidant, but it promotes the body's use of other key antioxidants—vitamins C and E, and CoQ10. It also stimulates the body's production of glutathione. Alpha-lipoic acid has been used in Europe to treat peripheral nerve degeneration and control blood sugar levels; it helps the body detoxify from heavy metal exposure and protects nerve tissues against oxidative stress. Some experts suggest 50 to 100 milligrams three times a day.

COENZYME Q10

Coenzyme Q10, known as CoQ10, is one of the antioxidants mentioned frequently in conjunction with Parkinson's disease and is considered by many practitioners as one of the most important supplements in a Parkinson's disease treatment protocol. CoQ10 is found in the mitochondria of cells and has a role in energy production and prevention of cellular death. Some research has found that the level of CoQ10 is substantially lower in the mitochondria of people with Parkinson's disease, and that a CoQ10 deficiency can increase the risk of dopamine cell death in the substantia nigra region of the brain. Taking CoQ10 improved energy production in cells. Practitioners recommend from 100 to 200 milligrams, two to four times daily, with meals. Results from a new study of CoQ10 in persons with Parkinson's disease should offer further understanding soon.

ACETYL-L-CARNITINE (ALC)

Acetyl-L-carnitine is an amino acid that has a role in transporting fatty acids into a cell's mitochondria, with the objective of producing energy. Some experts have claimed that acetyl-L-carnitine protects brain cells against aging-related degeneration and can improve mood, memory, and thinking. One study found that acetyl-L-carnitine could impact the brain's use of glucose, and even slow progression of Alzheimer's disease in younger patients, attesting to its neurological abilities. Practitioners frequently recommend 1,000 to 2,000 milligrams a day.

VINPOCETINE

Vinpocetine, a supplement derived from the periwinkle plant, has been used for several decades in Europe as a treatment for cerebrovascular disorders and senility symptoms. Vinpocetine's main functions are to aid in general circulation and blood flow to the brain, enhance the brain's utilization of oxygen, and reduce clotting in the brain, which can impair circulation. Other studies claim that vinpocetine can protect against neurological damage seen in aging. In various tests, vinpocetine was shown to measurably improve the functioning of elderly patients with chronic cerebral dysfunction and central nervous system degenerative disorders. Follow the label or your practitioner's instructions on when and how much to take.

OCTACOSANOL

Octacosanol is a lipid that comes from wheat-germ oil. Some practitioners recommend it to help increase endurance and to improve mood and daily living activities in Parkinson's disease. Follow the label or your practitioner's instructions on when and how much to take.

ESSENTIAL FATTY ACIDS

Essential fatty acids are a category of supplement that includes evening primrose oil, flax seeds, flaxseed oil, Udo's Oil, and other supplements. Essential fatty acids are often deficient in people with Parkinson's disease. Evening primrose oil—sometimes referred to as EPO—is of particular interest, because some studies have shown that after treatment with two teaspoons per day for several months, more than half of the patients studied had a reduction in tremor. A typical dosage of EPO is 1 tablespoonful (500 to 1,000 milligrams) twice daily.

EPA AND DHA

These are the omega 3s typically found in fish—sometimes known as "fish-oil supplements"—that are particularly known for their anti-inflammatory abilities. A typical dose is 300 to 400 milligrams per day of EPA or DHA, or a combination supplement.

FLAVONOIDS

The flavonoid supplements, and in particular those known as proanthocyanidins—which include grape seed extract and pine bark extract—are powerful antioxidants that can cross the blood-brain barrier, fighting free-radical damage and inflammation. By acting as free-radical scavengers, they could play a role in possibly preventing and slowing the progression of Parkinson's disease. Some practitioners suggest taking 25 to 50 milligrams of either three times daily.

NICOTINAMIDE ADENINE DINUCLEOTIDE HYDROGEN

Nicotinamide adenine dinucleotide hydrogen (NADH) is an enzyme that can aid in the function of the brain's neurotransmitters and may aid in raising the level of dopamine in the brain. Noted holistic physician Dr. Robert Atkins has had success with NADH for Parkinson's disease. In his book *Dr. Atkins' Vita-Nutrient Solution*, he indicates that Parkinson's patients have stopped trembling and have regained a steady gait on NADH. He also claims the supplement can create additional energy and may slow the deterioration of the nervous system. A review of four published studies using NADH for Parkinson's showed improvement in an open-labeled, non-placebo-controlled population, but no improvement in the one small placebo-controlled study that was conducted. Importantly, however, no adverse reactions were found with short-term oral or IV NADH use. NADH is considered most effective when administered intravenously, but testing of oral NADH has found that the formulation of one particular brand, Enada, may be most effective in pill form. Practitioners who recommend NADH typically suggest a dose of 5 to 20 milligrams twice daily.

PHOSPHATIDYL SERINE

Phosphatidyl serine is a type of lipid that plays a role in normal brain function and transmission of nerve impulses. Low levels of phosphatidyl serine have been linked to Parkinson's disease, and supplementation in Parkinson's patients has been shown to improve their mood and mental function. Dr. Robert Atkins recommends phosphatidyl serine for Parkinson's disease patients, to help the brain function properly and boost thinking, mood, and learning ability. In his book *Dr. Atkins' Vita-Nutrient Solution,* he recommends doses of 300 to 500 milligrams daily over a three-to-six-month period, to increase brain activity.

GINKGO BILOBA

Ginkgo biloba is a potent supplement that can help the body rid itself of free radicals, while enhancing circulation to the brain. It has been shown to be effective in improving memory, but ginkgo may also help with sleepiness or fatigue that is common in Parkinson's patients. Some experts, including Dr. Barbara Maddoux, believe that ginkgo biloba may be helpful for Parkinson's disease, because of its ability to help blood circulation in the brain. According to Dr. Maddoux:

Ginkgo biloba is very specific in supporting antioxidant activity in the brain, retina, and cardiovascular system. Studies have shown that it can enhance short- and long-term memory, improve circulation, and enhance concentration.

Some informal studies have suggested that in patients with Parkinson's disease, use of ginkgo could improve brain waves and appeared to increase brain metabolism. In 1997, researchers at the New York Institute for Medical Research reported on a clinical study of ginkgo biloba and dementia in the *Journal of the American Medical Association,* describing how 120 milligrams a day slowed cognitive decline in people with dementia. Some experts recommend starting at a dose of 120 milligrams a day and going up to 240 milligrams a day as needed. (Remember to talk to your doctor before using any ginkgo biloba, however, particularly if you are already taking blood circulation or blood-thinning drugs, as it can have additional blood-thinning properties.)

CHOLINE, LECITHIN, AND PHOSPHATIDYLCHOLINE

Some practitioners recommend that Parkinson's disease patients who have memory, thinking, or dementia symptoms should take a trio of memory-enhancing nutrients that include choline, lecithin, and phosphatidylcholine. All three of these supplements are precursors to acetylcholine—meaning that through chemical reactions, they are transformed into acetylcholine—which is one of the key neurotransmitters in the brain that move messages between brain cells. Experts advise taking these supplements early in the day to help maximize improvements in brain function throughout the day. Some experts recommend levels of 2,500 to 10,000 milligrams a day of choline, 10,000 to 15,000 grams a day of lecithin, and 1,200 to 6,000 milligrams a day of phosphatidylcholine.

MILK THISTLE

Milk thistle is an effective liver tonic that helps protect the liver from toxins and that can detoxify and rejuvenate a liver that is damaged by toxic exposure. In his book *The Brain Wellness Plan,* neurologist Dr. Jay Lombard advises Parkinson's disease patients who are taking any anti-Parkinson drugs to take 300 milligrams of standardized milk thistle daily.

ST. JOHN'S WORT

St. John's wort is a popular herbal supplement that works as an antidepressant in mild depression, acting similarly to the prescription serotonin reuptake inhibitors (SSRIs). For antidepressant effects, 300 milligrams three times daily is usually recommended. Note, however, that St. John's wort should not be used at the same time as other antidepressant medications—i.e., Prozac, Zoloft, Paxil, or other SSRIs. St. John's wort also interacts with some other prescription medications, so you should always discuss this supplement with your practitioner. St. John's wort is *not* considered an effective treatment for major depressive disorder.

GINGER

Ginger is an excellent remedy for nausea and vomiting, including stomach upset caused by medications. Fresh ginger root, available at most grocery stores, can be prepared in a liquid form, by covering a one-inch slice in water, bringing to a boil, and simmering for thirty minutes. Crystallized ginger is also an option. Easily obtained at natural foods stores, a small piece can be nibbled as needed.

Herbs and Other Supplements

A variety of herbs, flowers, and other supplements are also recommended for Parkinson's disease symptoms. It's best to consult a professional herbalist for advice regarding those herbs to take, and the appropriate dosage.

PASSIONFLOWER

Passionflower is a flower that is frequently recommended for Parkinson's patients. It was found to improve the effectiveness of levodopa and may reduce passive tremor. The flower contains two reportedly effective compounds that help with Parkinson's disease—harmine and harmaline alkaloids.

LADY'S SLIPPER

This herb is considered good for tremors, especially in more debilitated Parkinson's patients. It's also considered helpful for depression.

SKULLCAP

This herb can be combined with lady's slipper for greater strength and help in brain function. Experts advise tincture, 10–30 drops a day.

RHUBARD/PEONY/LICORICE/MAGNOLIA-BARK COMBINATION (WITH BUPLEURUM)

This combination of herbs is thought to help with tremors and relax stiff muscles. Sometimes bupleurum is added to aid in irritability, anxiety, and insomnia.

❖ SUPPLEMENT QUESTIONS AND CONTROVERSIES

Vitamin B$_6$

B$_6$ is a controversial vitamin for Parkinson's patients. Some experts caution that vitamin B$_6$ can interfere with levodopa and should not be taken. This was the case for patients taking levodopa alone before the mid-1970s, but other experts say that since that time, the switch to the use of carbidopa/levodopa combination drugs—and the obsolescence of the levodopa-only therapy—eliminates this concern over interaction. However, the mythology about the B$_6$-levodopa reaction is still mistakenly conveyed to patients taking carbidopa/levodopa. Currently, the reality is that Parkinson's disease patients may actually be deficient in vitamin B$_6$, which is needed in order to properly synthesize dopamine. Some researchers claim that supplementation with vitamin B$_6$ can reduce cramps, lessen rigidity, and tremors, and aid in walking. A study documented decreased cramps, rigidity, and tremors and improvement in 8 cases out of 19 in walking and bladder control. In another study, 5 out of 11 patients improved; and in another study, out of 90 cases, 9 percent had permanent improvement. Some experts advise that vitamin B$_6$ should be taken at the end of the day, after the last carbidopa/levodopa drugs are taken. Typically, 10 to 100 milligrams of vitamin B$_6$ is recommended daily.

L-tyrosine

The use of l-tyrosine by Parkinson's patients is a controversial topic. L-tyrosine is a direct precursor to levodopa—it chemically converts to levodopa. In theory, then, adding l-tyrosine might be an alternative to the use of carbidopa/levodopa drugs. Some experts have used l-tyrosine (at 100 milligrams per 2.2 pounds of body weight) as an alternative to levodopa/carbidopa, and claimed that some patients had good results along with fewer side effects than those taking the prescription drugs. This approach is highly controversial, however, and should only be attempted with a holistic physician who has expertise in nutritional approaches to Parkinson's disease. Supplemental use of l-tyrosine for Parkinson's disease patients taking carbidopa/levodopa is not recommended by many practitioners, due to concerns over the supplement's ability to interfere with the transport of dopamine into the brain.

5-Hydroxytryptophan

5-Hydroxytryptophan (5-HTP) is a powerful supplement that may be able to help alleviate depression in Parkinson's patients. There are a variety of warnings regarding 5-HTP, however, and Parkinson's patients should take it only under the guidance of an experienced practitioner. 5-HTP should not be taken on its own as a treatment for Parkinson's disease, but rather, along with a carbidopa/levodopa drug, because the supplement can worsen symptoms and, in particular, aggravate rigidity. For patients taking Eldepryl, 5-HTP should be taken only under the guidance and advice of a physician, as it can rarely cause dangerously high levels of serotonin and result in a serotinergic crisis.

SAMe

You'll need to consult with your practitioner regarding use of the popular supplement S-adenosylmethionine (SAMe), which is frequently used to treat for depression. Since some studies have suggested that SAMe may be able to block levodopa's effects, and others have suggested that it enhances levodopa's effects, there is no agreement on the interaction of this supplement with Parkinson's drugs. Discuss this with your physician before taking this supplement.

❖ WHAT WORKS

One patient who follows a vigorous schedule of aerobic exercise, yoga, t'ai chi, and stretching has also added supplements to her program. Says Bette:

> In addition to these exercises, I meditate and pray daily and take CoQ10, vitamins C and E, and beta-carotene. I still need to take medication for Parkinson's disease, but I really believe that combining alternative therapies with the medication offers me the best treatment. It gives me a sense of being able to impact my health by keeping my body as healthy as I can and not just relying on a pill to do that.

Marvin has had Parkinson's disease for ten years.

I used to just rely on taking the medicine my doctor prescribed for Parkinson's. Then my wife started reading about nutrition and antioxidants. I added a multivitamin, ginkgo biloba, CoQ10, grape seed extract, and extra vitamin C and E about four years ago. My energy level has improved; I have had less fatigue and less colds and respiratory infections. I can't really tell if the Parkinson's is better because of taking these, but it hasn't worsened much and I think my overall health is better by taking supplements. I feel good about taking an active role in my health and I am hopeful some of these might slow the progression of Parkinson's disease.

Jennifer had trouble with concentration, memory, and depression in addition to the motor symptoms of Parkinson's disease. She found that her memory, mood, and sleep improved a few weeks after starting St. John's wort. She then added ginkgo biloba and noted that her memory and thinking were sharper. Because she was able to feel better with these supplements, she did not need to take prescribed antidepressants.

It should always be remembered that if you do have serious, persistent signs and symptoms of depression, you may need prescription medicine. While herbs like St. John's wort may be helpful in the treatment of mild depression, they may not be effective for the treatment of major depression.

❖ GLUTATHIONE THERAPY

One special nutritionally oriented treatment that may be promising for Parkinson's patients is the use of intravenous (IV) glutathione. The theory behind this treatment is that glutathione, a naturally occurring brain chemical, is deficient in Parkinson's patients. As a brain antioxidant, glutathione's role in the brain is to protect against damage from free radicals. As we've seen before, one of the leading theories about what causes Parkinson's disease is that the presence of free radicals can injure dopamine cells and cause them to die. It's thought that glutathione can both help relieve symptoms of Parkinson's disease and perhaps help to prevent further damage to brain cells.

In the United States, this IV glutathione treatment for Parkinson's and neurological conditions has been pioneered by holistic physician David Perlmutter, M.D., a board-certified neurologist who runs the Perlmutter Health Center in Naples, Florida, and is the author of *BrainRecovery.com,* a book on nutritional support for brain conditions and health. Dr. Perlmutter began using intravenous glutathione as a treatment for Parkinson's disease in late 1998.

Dr. Perlmutter claims that IV glutathione can reduce the motor symptoms of Parkinson's disease and improve depression. According to Dr. Perlmutter, 80 percent of his patients trying IV glutathione have dramatically positive results with the treatment, and among those who try it, about 80 percent are still on the therapy a year after starting, enjoying continued improvements. However, it should be pointed out that most of these patients also need to take traditional medications to help control the motor symptoms of Parkinson's disease, in addition to their IV glutathione.

In addition to his own anecdotal experience with patients, Dr. Perlmutter points to an Italian study that claimed that a month of twice-daily intravenous glutathione therapy resulted in improvements for all patients and a 42 percent decline in disability overall.

Although these various observations are important to note, it's essential to clarify that to date, there are no published reports of placebo-controlled studies on the use of IV glutathione for the treatment of Parkinson's disease. These claims are based upon individual observations and therefore cannot be taken as proof that glutathione is truly helpful for the treatment of motor symptoms of Parkinson's disease or is neuroprotective, and at this time, it is not an accepted or recommended treatment for Parkinson's disease among most Parkinson's disease experts.

In his book *BrainRecovery.com,* Dr. Perlmutter cites anecdotal results, quoting from a letter from a physician with Parkinson's disease in his late fifties.

> I received my first dose of glutathione in your office that day, and within two hours I felt like a new person. I was more animated and expressive almost immediately. Over the next few weeks, my voice became stronger, I felt less tired, and my tremor almost disappeared. More slowly, my writing has improved. . . . My depression is gone and I have my sense of humor back.

One patient, Robby, was diagnosed over twenty years ago with Parkinson's disease. He had a pallidotomy six years ago with a definite improvement and is currently taking IV glutathione in addition to conventional Parkinson's drugs. Says Robby:

> I am hoping it will slow down or reverse the Parkinson's. I do think my movements are a little better and my muscles are less stiff since taking it.

Other patients have reported that IV glutathione didn't have the promised results. John, a Parkinson's disease patient for more than a decade, was interested in alternative therapies and tried IV glutathione.

> I tried IV glutathione therapy for up to eight straight months of daily injections. I finally stopped because I couldn't tell if it was doing anything for me—my Parkinson's disease symptoms didn't change at all. The glutathione therapy didn't hurt me in any way, but it didn't seem to help.

At present, the main medical evidence in support of the IV glutathione therapy is still anecdotal. But some reputable Parkinson centers believe, in theory, that it may be a valid treatment for Parkinson's disease and is worth investigation with scientifically controlled studies. One such center is the University of Miami. The NPF Center of Excellence there, under the direction of Dr. William Koller and Dr. Kelly Lyons, has planned a randomized crossover double-blinded study of twenty Parkinson's disease patients. Initially, ten will receive placebo and ten will receive IV glutathione for one month, and then, following a two-week period with no treatment or placebo, each patient will receive the other treatment for an additional month. The standard Unified Parkinson Disease Rating Scale (UPDRS) will be performed. This scale helps to measure PD motor symptoms, and each patient will be rated before starting treatment and after one month and two months to determine whether they improve in their motor function while receiving glutathione more than when receiving placebo. It is important that controlled studies like this are performed in order to more critically evaluate whether IV glutathione is beneficial for persons with Parkinson's disease.

IV glutathione also requires a doctor's prescription and supervision. While IV glutathione is FDA-approved as a nutritional supplement, it is not an approved Parkinson's disease treatment. For use in Parkinson's disease, Dr. Perlmutter has found that the optimal dose is 1,400 milligrams, three times a week, delivered in a ten-minute treatment. According to Dr. Perlmutter, while initial treatments are done in a physician's office, a patient's caregiver can be taught to perform the procedure so that treatments can take place more conveniently at home.

It would be unusual for patients with moderate to severe Parkinson's disease to go off their Parkinson's medicines and use IV glutathione alone and have sufficient control of their motor symptoms. Therefore, the treatment is typically done alongside prescribed Parkinson's medications, such as carbidopa/levodopa. Dr. Perlmutter claims that, over time, however, some of his patients may need a dosage reduction of their conventional medications after being on glutatione therapy for Parkinson's disease.

Dr. Perlmutter believes that the treatment is safe, and reports that he has seen almost no side effects among his patients, except one patient had a niacin-like flush, and one or two who had headaches.

Despite Dr. Perlmutter's views, many physicians are unwilling to prescribe IV glutathione because it is not yet a proven treatment for Parkinson's disease. In addition, the treatment requires frequent IV injections, which carries an increased risk of infection. As with many alternative therapies, the cost is also typically not currently covered under most insurance plans.

◈ CHELATION

Chelation refers to the process of drawing out excess metals from the bloodstream and organs. In chelation therapy, chelating agents or herbs chemically bind to and attach themselves to metals such as lead, arsenic, mercury, cadmium, and aluminum in the bloodstream. The metals are then flushed out of the body via normal processes of elimination, such as urination. Typically, practitioners recommend multiple treatments over time in order to achieve optimal results.

Chelation therapy is most frequently done as an intravenous therapy, in which a certain amino acid complex called EDTA (ethylene-diamine-tetra-acetic acid) is given over a several-hour period.

While the intravenous method is considered the most effective, there are some specialized herbs and supplements—such as marine alginate concentrate and N-acetylcysteine, for example—that can be used for chelation. Some nutritionally oriented practitioners can advise regarding a customized IV or supplement-based chelation program.

Since research has found that many Parkinson's patients have an increased level of iron in those areas of the brain that are usually damaged by the condition, it's thought that chelation may be a helpful treatment for ridding the body of excess iron. The theory is that removing overloads of toxic metals lowers the immune response against these toxins and also helps in reducing production of harmful free radicals. Cell energy increases, and cells can rebuild and regenerate more easily.

Chelation is considered a safe treatment, but needs to be determined and administered by an expert practitioner. As in the case of many of these alternative therapies, controlled studies for the treatment of Parkinson's disease with chelation therapy have not been performed, and among traditional Parkinson disease specialists this is not a recommended treatment for Parkinson's disease.

❖ HORMONE SUPPLEMENTATION

While it does not specifically fall into the category of nutrition, hormone supplementation is important to touch upon for Parkinson's patients, because hormonal balance is required for both optimal energy in brain cells and optimal brain function.

Estrogen and Testosterone

One important area to evaluate, particularly if you are having cognitive symptoms or dementia, is hormonal balance. Hormonal imbalances—whether related to or separate from the Parkinson's disease—may have an impact on cognitive function and dementia symptoms. In women, a drop in estrogen levels, for example, frequently causes well-known symptoms such as hot flashes, sleep disturbances, and vaginal dryness, but can also cause major mood swings, fatigue, and memory problems. Low testosterone in women can cause low sex drive. In women, insufficient progesterone can also cause symptoms such as fatigue and depression. In men, a drop in testosterone levels can cause muscle loss, high cholesterol, reduced sex drive, and depression and memory changes. Blood tests can evaluate estrogen, testosterone, and progesterone levels, and supplementation, by prescription patches, gels, creams, pills, or injection, can help restore proper balance and relieve hormone-deficiency–related symptoms.

Pregnenolone and DHEA

Dehydroepiandrosterone (DHEA) and its precursor, pregnenolone, are thought to improve the activity of brain cells and enhance memory. DHEA is a steroid hormone naturally produced by the body, and production drops substantially with age. Some experts theorize that pregnenolone and DHEA can help memory, relieve depression, create a sense of increased physical and psychological well-being, and protect neurological function. Practitioners typically recommend 50 to 150 milligrams a day of pregnenolone—taken in three equal doses—and 25 to 50 milligrams of DHEA a day. Women usually require less DHEA than men, so they typically remain in the lower end of the range.

Melatonin

Melatonin is a hormone that is produced by the brain's pineal gland when you are sleeping in total darkness. Melatonin is thought to have a role in stimulating the synthesis of serotonin, and can be a help to some Parkinson's patients in terms of enhancing cognitive function. Melatonin is typically taken in doses of 500 micrograms to 3 milligrams a night, usually an hour before bedtime.

❖ CONCLUSION

Clearly, good nutrition, healthy diet, and proper use of vitamin and other supplements can positively impact an individual's health. Whether any of the above treatments can slow the progress of Parkinson's disease or dramatically lessen its motor symptoms remains largely unknown. To date, most of these therapies have not been formally studied with placebo-controlled, blinded studies in people with Parkinson's disease. That is why it is important to remind readers that the information in this chapter should not be considered as accepted, proven treatments for Parkinson's disease. Rather, consider them talking points for exploration under the guidance and direction of licensed nutritionists, dieticians, herbalists, M.D.s, D.O.s, and D.O.M.s. Certainly, these therapies can help alleviate or lessen many physical symptoms and enhance or restore the body's physiological functions and promote good physical and mental health, and as more studies are completed, we may find even more proven benefits.

Part IV

LIVING WITH PARKINSON'S DISEASE

Chapter 9

Additional Help for Persistent Symptoms

My hands may tremble but my heart does not.
—*Janet Reno*

Even when you are receiving the best possible Parkinson's disease treatment from your health care team, you may have persistent symptoms that interfere with your ability to function on a day-to-day basis. But there are solutions worth considering that can help minimize—or even eliminate—some of the more common persistent health challenges.

◈ DYSKINESIA

One of the most bothersome symptoms for Parkinson's patients is dyskinesia, the term used to describe irregular writhing, dancelike movements. If fast, these movements are called chorea; if slower, are called athetosis; and if very slowed, with posturing of a limb, neck, or trunk, are called dystonia.

Dyskinesia is not actually a symptom of Parkinson's disease. Rather, it is a side effect from long-term use of carbidopa/levodopa and can sometimes result from use of the dopamine agonist drugs. One recent study reported that a review of the medical literature over the past thirty-four years found that one-third of Parkinson's patients developed dyskinesia four to six years after starting carbidopa/levodopa therapy, and almost 90 percent developed dyskinesia after nine or more years.

Treatment of dyskinesia typically involves adjustment of the medications used to treat Parkinson's disease. In cases where dyskinesia is severe and medication adjustments have failed to work, surgical treatment with either pallidotomy or deep brain stimulation can be very beneficial, by reducing the amount of dyskinesia up to 90 percent.

Treatment approaches to lessen dyskinesia include the following:

- Lower the dose of carbidopa/levodopa.
- Add a dopamine agonist to carbidopa/levodopa.
- Change from carbidopa/levodopa CR/ER form to the immediate-release form.
- Add Symmetrel (amantadine).
- Lower the dose of carbidopa/levodopa and add a COMT inhibitor.
- Consider surgery (DBS or pallidotomy).

Jerry describes his experiences with dyskinesia that led him to pursue surgery.

When it was so bad, I would lie down on the floor and put my head between the couch and wall and try to tense all my muscles to make it stop. Sometimes it would last five hours like that. Once I had a bad attack in the car—my wife, Donna, was driving and I was in the front passenger seat and my body was so out of control that my legs kept banging up against the windshield until I cracked it. That was it—I decided at that moment something had to change. Life just wasn't worth living.

Linda talks about her battle against dyskinesia:

I had such good control of my tremors and could move almost normally when I took my medicine for Parkinson's, but then a couple of years after starting Sinemet, I started to have jerky movement of my arms and legs. It usually happened about an hour after I took my medicine and sometimes would last three hours. It got so bad at times that I couldn't use my arms or legs, I would just jerk all over. I felt like I was possessed. It was so much worse than the tremors and slowness. My doctor lowered the dose of Sinemet by half and the movements stopped, but I became too slow and my tremors came back. Then my doctor added Permax and I could move better with less tremor, but this time with very little dyskinesia, only a little wiggle here and there.

❖ SPEAKING AND SWALLOWING PROBLEMS

The majority of people with Parkinson's disease have some form of speech problems, even with drug treatment. Some of the more common challenges include

• A reduction in the vocal volume;
• A voice that fades out as you keep talking;

- Monotonous pitch that lacks expressiveness or changes in tone;
- Hoarse or breathy speaking voice;
- Poor articulation, with slurring;
- Rapid speaking, running together words without stopping; and
- Hesitation when beginning to speak or starting sentences.

The key with speaking problems is to work on them as soon as they appear. If you work with a conventional speech therapist or pathologist as soon as speech difficulties appear, you can learn exercises to deal with these various concerns, and help minimize further worsening of speech problems. But once speech problems are substantial, therapy can only help to some extent. Speech therapists may also focus on exercises for breathing, and tongue, lip, and jaw exercises. These can all help with loudness of the voice and also help correct some respiratory problems.

A special type of speech therapy is known as the "Lee Silverman Voice Treatment." This treatment, which is offered by trained speech-language pathologists, involves sixteen sessions over a four-week period and teaches patients how to produce a louder voice, increase intelligibility of speech, and modulate volume by exercising and controlling voice box muscles. In some studies, Parkinson's disease patients who have this treatment were able to improve voice volume, tone, and quality and to maintain those improvements as much as two years after treatment. Further information can be obtained by contacting the Lee Silverman Voice Treatment Foundation, at 888-606-LSVT (5788), or via their Web site, http://www.lsvt.org/.

Collagen injections are another option when there is vocal cord weakness contributing to speech problems. Collagen is a particular type of protein that is found underneath the skin. For this treatment, collagen is harvested either from cows or from the patient. Once an allergy test shows that there is no allergy to collagen, the fifteen-minute procedure can be provided. Treatment involves application of a spray anesthetic to throat and nostril. A thin, flexible tube is inserted into the nose and down the throat, allowing for a view of the vocal cords. A syringe containing the collagen is inserted through the side of the neck, and the collagen is injected into the vocal cords.

Collagen injections work by increasing the size of the vocal cords, so that the vocal cords that have been slowed by the Parkinson's become fatter and closer together, which makes them more effective at generating sound.

One patient, Phil, had Parkinson's disease for eight years, and voice problems began three years after diagnosis. Although his medicines helped to effectively control his tremors and slowness, his most disabling symptom—hypophonia—did not respond to the medicines he was prescribed. Phil complained that his voice was often so quiet that others found it hard to understand him when sitting even three feet away, and rarely was he able to effectively communicate via telephone. After researching online, Phil found an ear, nose, and throat specialist who was skilled at performing collagen injections into vocal cords for treatment of this problem. Says Phil:

> After suffering with this for five years, I was anxious to go forward with the procedure. Within a week after the injections, I had a dramatic improvement in the volume of my voice. People can now hear me. I still have a little difficulty on the phone at times, but overall I'm delighted with the improvement.

Vocal cord implants are another option, when someone has lost their voice due to weakened vocal cords. The FDA-approved implants add volume to a weakened vocal cord by pushing it to the center of the voice box, where it can more effectively produce sound. The half-hour procedure, which is done with local anesthesia, involves the doctor testing particular devices in the vocal cord area, via a small opening made through the thyroid cartilage. The patient tests out his or her voice with each testing device, until the voice is identified by the patient as normal, and then the tester is removed and a same-size implant is inserted.

Some patients opt to use computer communication boards or a handheld microphone to amplify their voice rather than consider a surgical procedure that is not fully guaranteed to work.

Some patients with more advanced Parkinson's disease can have difficulties with swallowing, evidenced by coughing, gagging, or choking on food. Speech therapists trained in swallowing disorders can help evaluate the situation and recommend solutions and techniques to help minimize the problem. Patients with persistent problems may also benefit from a swallow study and examination by a speech therapist and possibly a referral to a gastroenterologist, who may be able to evaluate and recommend additional treatments. Very rarely, people who have severe swallowing problems and recurrent secondary aspiration pneumonia or malnourishment may need to consider placement of a feeding tube (PEG tube) directly into the stomach. This is more commonly needed in progressive supranuclear palsy (PSP), one of the Parkinson-Plus syndromes.

◆ FREEZE ATTACKS

Freezing, a temporary inability to move, occurs in an estimated 30 percent of Parkinson's patients, usually later in the course of the condition. It's more common in those patients whose Parkinson's started out with problems related to walking and balance.

The times when freezing is most likely to occur include

- When getting up from a chair or bed and starting to walk;
- When approaching a doorway or walking through a doorway;
- When going into a tight space or elevator;
- When going up and down steps or over curbs; and
- When turning.

The key to dealing with a freeze attack is to break the freeze, particularly before you might lose your balance and risk a fall.

Some people find that what helps them is developing their own set of prompts or triggers for walking. Some tricks can be used to help break a freeze:

- Imagine a line (i.e., a line of tape or a painted finish line) on the floor, then try to step over it.
- Hum or imagine a marching tune or count rhythmically to yourself.
- Aim for tiles or marks on the floor.
- Place dark-colored adhesive tape on the floor to make lines to step over.
- Step over your partner's foot.
- Rock from side to side to get started.

One technique that helps some people is to create visual markers in frequently traveled paths in the home. For example, marking frequently traveled routes such as from the living room to the kitchen, or from the bedroom to the bathroom, creates visual cues and markers that can help with freezing or hesitation.

If someone is there, have him or her put a foot in front of you so that you can step over it, or have them tap you on the shoulder, or ask them to give you a hand to help.

For freeze attacks, canes can also be fitted with a "step-over," which is a plastic attachment that extends out from the bottom of the cane and can serve as a visual cue, or with a drop-down lever that drops on the foot and may release a freeze.

One device that patients have found helpful with freezing is a special cane that is equipped with a laser pointer. In one research study, patients with Parkinson's were tested, and told to point the laser in the direction they wanted to move, and then to focus on stepping on the beam. Most of the subjects showed significant improvements in mobility. Other studies have found that frequent use of a laser pointer may make the benefits less effective over time.

Adjusting medicines may help in some patients, to ensure proper dosage and proper timing of dosage to maximize "on"-time and minimize "off"-times.

Some Parkinson's disease patients have found that trained companion dogs can help with walking and, in particular, freezing. With freezing, patients can't continue or initiate movement without some sort of physical cue. Companion dogs can be trained to actually provide this triggering cue, by tapping on a patient's foot with their paws. Dogs can also help open doors, retrieve lost objects, and help with balance, and help patients get back up after a fall. Working with a well-trained dog can reduce falls from 75 to 80 percent, according to research reported on in the National Parkinson Foundation's *Parkinson Report.*

While some Parkinson's patients are encouraged to get walkers, new research presented to the American Neurological Association in late 2001 found that walking aids such as walkers do not solve the problem of freezing. In research, Dr. Christopher Goetz of Rush Presbyterian–St. Luke's Medical Center in Chicago had nineteen Parkinson's patients follow an obstacle course. Dr. Goetz found that both standard and wheeled walkers slowed down the patients, and those patients using the walkers also had more freezing.

❖ PREVENTING FALLS

Falls typically occur when Parkinson's disease symptoms affect balance. When balance becomes unsteady, the ability to react is delayed, and stiffness and rigidity set in, reaction time can be affected, and falls can result.

The most vulnerable times for falls include

- When getting up from a chair;
- When sitting down in a chair;
- With the first step when starting to walk;
- When turning while walking; and
- When stepping on or off a curb or stair.

Walkers, particularly rolling walkers that have wheels, can be a help to some patients. However, some patients have a more difficult time with wheeled walkers, as they can go too fast and contribute to falling. If that occurs, removing the wheels and placing tennis balls on the ends of the four pegs will allow the person to slowly push the walker on a hard floor or firm carpet. In addition, some of the new large wheeled walkers have hand brakes and a seat so that the person can sit and rest when needed.

Canes, both standard and quad (with four legs that can stand on their own), can be a help to some people with walking. The benefit to a quad cane is that it's always standing ready at chairside or bedside and is more stable.

High-heeled shoes can be a problem. Some practitioners believe the ideal shoe is a high-top sneaker, which provides better balance and ankle support. Also, if you tend to shuffle, you might want to switch to leather-soled shoes. They can be less sticky and are less likely to cause you to stumble than rubber soles.

Physical therapy from a therapist who specializes in balance can help improve posture and teach a Parkinson's patient to use arms for balance and to take bigger steps—all techniques that can reduce the risk of falling.

Exercise—in particular, treadmill walking—can help strengthen legs, reduce stiffness, and help with general mobility. T'ai chi and yoga exercises that focus on centering one's balance can be very helpful to improve balance and make body movements more efficient.

All people with Parkinson's disease should safety-proof their homes by removing throw rugs or any obstacles and installing grab bars and railings near the toilet, shower, bed, and stairs. Use of shower chairs and handheld detachable showerheads may be a great benefit for those who have difficulty with balance. Also, simple changes in behavior, such as remembering to be seated when doing things like dressing, can prevent unnecessary falls.

◈ SKIN CHANGES

Seborrheic dermatitis and dandruff, which are frequent side effects of Parkinson's disease, can sometimes easily be treated by dandruff shampoos that contain salicylic acid and coal tars. Over-the-counter 1 percent hydrocortisone cream applied to the affected areas may greatly lessen flaking and itching of the scalp and forehead. Other prescription medicines such as ammonium lactate (Lac-Hydrin) may be helpful. If these therapies do not work, then consultation with a dermatologist should be sought.

◈ HYPOTENSION, LIGHT-HEADEDNESS, AND FAINTING

A lowering of blood pressure upon standing can occur as a side effect from all of the medicines used to treat Parkinson's disease, as well as from many blood pressure medicines, some antidepressants, and drugs used to treat bladder dysfunction. A review and adjustment of one's medicines and evaluation by a cardiologist to rule out heart problems should be considered for recurrent fainting or near-fainting spells. Simple treatments to reduce light-headedness and near fainting include wearing support stockings, slowly rising from a lying or sitting position, placing blocks under the head of the bed, adding salt to one's diet (if okayed by your doctor), and adding caffeinated beverages or over-the-counter tablets. Prescription drugs that can help treat fainting that results from lowering of blood pressure include fludrocortisone (Florinef), midodrine (Proamatine), and indomethacin (Indocine).

◆ EXCESSIVE SALIVA AND DROOLING (SIALORRHEA)

Excessive drooling may be reduced by taking carbidopa/levodopa (Sinemet), dopamine agonists, and anticholinergic agents (Artane and Cogentin). In people who do not have a history or symptoms of heart disease, placing a few drops of atropine ophthalmic 1 percent solution on a spoon and then adding tap water and swishing and swallowing before bedtime may reduce nighttime and daytime drooling. In addition, injection of botulinum toxin into the salivary glands may be helpful in severe cases of sialorrhea.

◆ CONSTIPATION

Constipation, which is defined as having fewer bowel movements than usual, with a long or hard passing of stools, is very common in Parkinson's disease. Anti-Parkinson drugs can cause constipation, so you should review your medicines with your physician. Remember that there is no "right" number of daily or weekly bowel movements. "Regularity" may mean bowel movements twice a day for some people or just twice a week for others. But if it's determined that you are having constipation, there are a variety of things you can do to help deal with this situation.

- Drink enough water. You absolutely need to, at minimum, drink eight 8-ounce glasses of water-based, caffeine-free beverages. That could be water, caffeine-free herbal tea, or unsweetened seltzers.
- Increase the amount of fiber in your diet. Fiber is also beneficial in helping speed up the response to levodopa. You can add fiber by increasing your intake of fresh fruits and

vegetables, either cooked or raw, as well as whole-grain cereals and breads. Dried fruit such as apricots, prunes, and figs are especially high in fiber.

- Avoid high-fat meats, dairy products, sugary desserts, and excess consumption of eggs or convenience foods, which can all contribute to constipation.

- Don't misuse laxatives or enemas. You may think of them as treatments for constipation, but laxatives and enemas should be used only on the advice of your physician, as they can be habit forming. If you rely on laxatives or enemas for too long, you may lose further bowel function and come to require them for elimination.

- Don't ignore the urge to have a bowel movement. While you may prefer to have your bowel movements at home, waiting can worsen chronic constipation.

- Be as active as possible. Physical activity helps contribute to normal bowel function, so get as much exercise or walking in as you possibly can.

- Consider adding bran to your diet. Unprocessed bran, also known as miller's bran, can be added to baked goods, cereals, and fruit. If you add bran, introduce it slowly, as it can cause some bloating and gas while your digestive system adjusts.

- Another remedy is also absolutely worth mentioning here. A basic and classic Ayurvedic herbal remedy known as triphala has been found to help digestion and constipation problems. Various triphala preparations are available at many natural health and vitamin stores, but a particularly reliable brand is Planetary Formulas Triphala.

If all of the above remedies have failed to regulate your bowel movements, you might try over-the-counter bulk agents like psyllium (Metamucil), methylcellulose (Citrucel), or docusate (Colace). These may need to be taken at twice the recommended dose in persons with Parkinson's disease in order to be effective. If this fails, then a prescription medication such as Lactulose or Miralax may be very effective in relieving constipation.

◈ INCONTINENCE

Incontinence refers to either the inability to hold urine or feces until you reach a toilet, or leakage due to stress or overflow.

If you are experiencing incontinence, you may try to hide the problem from friends, family, and even your doctor. But there are many options to treat and control, even cure the situation, so you need to speak up and bring this to the attention of your physician. This discussion and medical assessment by your doctor should be your first step. The doctor may refer you to a urologist, a doctor who specializes in diseases of the urinary tract, or to a gynecologist, a specialist in the female reproductive system.

There are some things that can be done to help treat incontinence:

- Behavioral techniques such as exercises for pelvic muscles, biofeedback, and training the bladder to control urination can help you wait until you can reach a toilet.
- Some medicines can be prescribed that treat incontinence, including oxybutinin (Ditropan), tolterodine tartrate (Detrol), and prazosin (Hytrin).
- Sometimes surgery can improve or cure incontinence if it is caused by a structural problem such as an abnormally positioned bladder or a prostate enlargement.

- Another option for serious and persistent bladder problems is what's known as a bladder pacemaker. This device is surgically implanted under the skin, in the lower-abdomen area. A wire containing electrodes is inserted at the base of the spine, near the nerves that regulate bladder function. The pacemaker sends painless electrical signals to the bladder to contract or relax as urine is stored or eliminated. In clinical trials, the pacemaker reduced leakage in 74 percent of patients within six months, and almost 50 percent of patients had no accidents or leakage at all.

When incontinence cannot be cured, there are some techniques to help manage the situation. For example, special absorbent pads can be used. Also, absorbent and even disposable underclothing, no more bulky than regular underwear, can be worn under your clothing. Also, in some cases, a flexible tube, known as an indwelling catheter, may be a solution. The catheter is inserted into the urethra, and urine is collected in a container. Men also can use an external collecting device that is fitted over the penis and is connected to a drainage bag, called a condom catheter. This can be very helpful for men who need to urinate frequently at night.

Although Parkinson's disease and its effect on the autonomic nervous system can cause incontinence, this problem can also occur as a side effect of some medicines or as a symptom of a bladder or urinary tract infection. (A sign of infection would be burning pain upon urination and possibly an unpleasant odor to the urine.) If you have difficulty with your bladder function, review all of your medications to be sure they are not the cause or contributing to your symptoms. Your physician can easily rule out an infection by checking a culture with a clean urine sample, and a urologist can perform an exam and tests to check for enlarged prostate or bladder pro-lapse, which can sometimes be the cause of these symptoms.

❖ SEXUAL DIFFICULTIES

Problems with sexual function may also occur as part of Parkinson's disease, resulting from the disruption of normal function of the autonomic nerves that regulate sexual function of the body. This is very common and probably vastly under-reported, due to the sensitive nature of the subject. Sexuality is a vital part of everyone's life and should be addressed and taken seriously, like all symptoms. If you are having a decrease in your sex drive or have the desire but cannot fully achieve and maintain an erection or reach orgasm, discuss your concerns with your physician. Your physician can evaluate you further to rule out other illnesses and conditions that can cause sexual problems, such as diabetes, hypothyroidism, poor blood circulation, hormonal imbalances, and depression. Your family doctor can perform simple blood tests to check for some of these and might refer you to a urologist or gynecologist for further evaluation. A long list of medicines can cause impotence, including some blood pressure medicines, especially beta-blockers, anticholinergics (Artane, Cogentin), sedatives, antianxiety and antidepressant agents, and antihistamines, among many others. Your physician can evaluate your medicines to determine if any of them may be contributing to sexual problems. It's also important to note that alcohol in excessive amounts can cause impotence.

Impotence may be effectively treated with a variety of medicines such as sildenafil (Viagra), which is very effective for men with Parkinson's disease, and possibly for women as well. One note of caution: Viagra should not be used in men or women who have serious active heart disease or who are taking nitrates. Other oral medications that can reduce impotence include yohimbine (Yocon) and bromocriptine (Parlodel), if prolactin levels are elevated. Injections directly into the penis with papaverine HCL (Papaverine), phentolamine (Regitine), or alprostadil (Caverject) may improve erections in 65 percent of all men regardless of the cause of impotence.

◈ FATIGUE AND SLEEP PROBLEMS

Fatigue is a common problem with Parkinson's patients. In some cases, the fatigue is actually from medications being taken. One study, conducted by Dr. Mahyar Etminan from the University of Toronto, found that patients who take ropinirole (Requip) and pramipexole (Mirapex) have a five times greater risk of sleepiness, compared with those taking placebo drugs. Patients are also more at risk of sudden "sleep attacks," in which extreme sleepiness comes on rapidly. The sleepiness that came from these drugs also put some patients more at risk of automobile accidents. The researchers said that physicians should make their patients aware of this side effect and advise patients who feel drowsy while taking ropinirole or pramipexole not to drive.

Frequently, however, the fatigue is either just a side effect of the condition overall, or the result of aging-related disturbances that are exacerbated by the Parkinson's disease. Insomnia is one of the most common complaints about sleep. Insomnia can refer to taking too long a time to fall asleep—i.e., more than thirty to forty-five minutes—or waking up many times each night. Insomnia can also include waking up early and being unable to get back to sleep, and waking up feeling tired.

If you are having insomnia, one of the first things you need to have evaluated is whether you may have sleep apnea. Apnea is a common problem that causes your breathing to stop for periods of up to two minutes, often many times each night. Apnea can be due to some sort of obstruction—air can't flow in or out of the nose or mouth—which is called obstructive apnea. Or, it can be central apnea, which is less common, and takes place when the brain doesn't send proper signals to start the breathing muscles. The combination of daytime sleepiness and loud snoring at night is a sign that you might have sleep apnea and should see a physician specializing in sleep disorders. Treatments for apnea include a change in sleeping position, devices to keep the airways open with supplemental oxygen at night, medication, and surgery.

When insomnia is not due to apnea, it can be helped by a variety of approaches.

- First, try to follow a regular sleeping schedule, going to sleep and getting up at the same time.
- Keep daytime naps to a minimum.
- Get regular exercise daily.
- Expose yourself to natural afternoon sunlight every day.
- Don't drink caffeinated beverages late in the day or evening.
- Avoid drinking alcohol late in the day or evening.
- Create a safe and comfortable place to sleep. The room should be dark, well-ventilated, and quiet.
- Develop a bedtime routine, which could include reading, a bath, or other relaxing activity.
- Use your bedroom only for sleeping.

If these techniques don't work, and you suffer insomnia for more than several weeks, it's time to discuss options with your practitioner. Natural or holistic practitioners may advise the use of melatonin or the herb kava kava as a sleep aid. Conventional practitioners have a variety of sleep-inducing drugs that may be of help to Parkinson's patients.

Older Parkinson's patients should be particularly careful about over-the-counter sleep aids that contain the drug diphenhydramine as an active ingredient, however. Products such as Sominex and Benadryl contain diphenhydramine, and researchers have found that the ingredient dramatically increases the risk of symptoms of delirium and dementia in patients age 70 or older. These may be very effective in younger persons, however. Tylenol PM is a fairly safe drug and may help one to sleep better. Sometimes it is necessary to add a short-acting sedative prescription medication (i.e., Ambien, Ativan).

Another common cause of sleep disturbance in Parkinson's patients is "restless legs syndrome" (RLS). This syndrome can cause crawly, prickly sensations, primarily in the legs, but sometimes affecting the arms and trunk. These sensations are more common and severe at night, are usually relieved by moving the legs, and can cause legs to jerk involuntarily during sleep—and sometimes even when awake. RLS may make it hard to fall asleep or may wake you up frequently.

Besides the recommendations for better sleep offered earlier in this section, the main drug treatments offered for restless legs syndrome are the dopamine-receptor agonist drugs, such as pramipexole (Mirapex), pergolide (Permax), and ropinirole (Requip), but also carbidopa/levodopa. Sedatives, such as the mild tranquilizer clonazepam (Klonopin), can be effective as nighttime treatments in some people. In people who have ongoing RLS, some doctors recommend pain relievers, such as propoxyphene (Darvon), oxycodone (Percocet), or hydrocodone (Vicodin). Anticonvulsants, in particular neurontin (Gabapentin), are also used in some patients who have extensive daytime symptoms and pain associated with their RLS.

❖ DEPRESSION

Everyone feels a bit down here and there, but when having a case of the blues persists, and interferes with your ability to function, then it's time to take a look at whether or not you might have clinical depression.

Symptoms of depression include the following:

- Persistent sad, anxious, or "empty" mood
- Feelings of hopelessness, pessimism
- Feelings of guilt, worthlessness, helplessness
- Loss of interest or pleasure in hobbies and activities that were once enjoyed, including sex
- Decreased energy, fatigue, being "slowed down"
- Difficulty concentrating, remembering, making decisions
- Insomnia, early-morning awakening, or oversleeping
- Appetite and/or weight loss or overeating and weight gain
- Thoughts of death or suicide; suicide attempts
- Restlessness, irritability
- Persistent physical symptoms that do not respond to treatment, such as headaches, digestive disorders, and chronic pain

Unfortunately, many of these symptoms may be dismissed—even by you, your doctor, family members, or a caretaker—as symptoms of "old age" or may be assumed to go along with the Parkinson's disease. But clinical depression can occur at any age and can exist alongside but separate from Parkinson's disease, so if you have these symptoms, you should talk to your doctor about being evaluated for depression.

Long-term, clinical depression may require antidepressant therapy (i.e., nortriptyline [Pamelor], sertraline [Zoloft], paroxetine [Paxil], citralopram [Celexa], venlafaxine [Effexor], mirtazapine [Remeron], or bupropion [Welbutrin]) in combination with talk therapy or psychotherapy. In cases of severe, catatonic depression, admission to the hospital and possible treatment with electroconvulsive therapy in addition to antidepressant medicine may be necessary. Milder depression can frequently respond to therapy, aerobic exercise, support groups, and herbal supplements, such as St. John's wort.

But the critical first step is to admit that help is needed. Mental illness is an uncomfortable topic for some people, and some people mistakenly believe that it is a sign of weakness to ask for mental health help and that one should be able to just "snap out of it" when depressed. But depression is a physical problem and deserves medical attention, not embarrassment. The first step in dealing with depression is a discussion with your general-practice or primary care doctor—which may be your neurologist—for an assessment. The doctor will evaluate for any other medical or drug-related causes for depression and should conduct a complete review of the medicines you are taking, along with blood tests for thyroid function (thyroid panel), a complete blood count (CBC), and a check of your vitamin B_{12} level. The doctor can then make a referral to a mental health specialist—i.e., a therapist, counselor, psychologist, or even one of a new type of specialist, a geriatric psychiatrist—for further assessment and treatment.

◆ WRITING PROBLEMS

The medicines used to treat Parkinson's disease usually help to improve micrographia (small and/or illegible handwriting). In addition to medication, there are various approaches you can take to help with this problem.

First, some people find that specialized occupational therapy geared toward writing and manipulating objects by hand can be of help.

Specialty stores and online outlets also sell a variety of writing aids, including special extra-wide "fat" pens and pens with special grips that make them easier to hold and write with.

Some people can obtain similar results by putting rubber bands on pens to make them fatter and easier to grip. If you have difficulty signing your name, you can ask your local bank to make a signature stamp for you that you can legally use for signing your checks.

Finally, some people have found that a computer, typewriter, or handheld pointer-input device—such as a Palm Pilot handheld computer—may be easier than handwriting for some tasks.

Inexpensive and effective voice-activation software can even make "typing" easier for those with limited dexterity or typing skills.

Kim found some simple solutions to her handwriting problems:

> I love to write letters and especially send out Christmas cards to all my friends, but found this to be an almost impossible task after being diagnosed with Parkinson's disease. My doctor increased the dose of my medicine and this helped a little, but the combination of Parkin-

son's and arthritis still hampered my writing. I found it much easier to type than to write, so I typed a letter for Christmas and had it copied and put in personal cards with just my signature. I am learning how to use my new computer and know how to e-mail my friends and how to look up information on the Internet about Parkinson's, so having problems with writing has taught me a lot.

❖ DEMENTIA, MEMORY, AND COGNITION

Memory loss is a problem for some Parkinson's patients. In the past, this was written off as a sign of aging, but it's now known that severe memory loss and confusion are not a normal part of aging. While some memory lapses or slowness in remembering certain details can be fairly benign and is somewhat common in Parkinson's disease, some patients will have more significant changes in memory, personality, and behavior that are characterized as dementia. The term *dementia* describes various symptoms that include repeating the same questions, becoming lost in familiar places, inability to follow directions, being disoriented, and neglecting safety, hygiene, and nutrition.

If you are concerned about memory and cognitive problems, your first step is to visit your primary care doctor or neurologist, for a complete medical examination to assess any identifiable causes. Be sure to review all of the medicine you are taking, because many medicines, including the ones for Parkinson's, can cause mental slowing and confusion. Virtually all of the medicines that are used to treat Parkinson's disease can cause side effects of mental dulling, confusion, and even hallucinations. Although carbidopa/levodopa (Sinemet) and the dopamine agonists can do this, the more notorious medicines that should be tapered off and stopped in cases of dementia with Parkinson's disease are the anticholinergics (trihexyphenidyl [Artane], benztropine mesylate [Cogentin], amantadine [Symmetrel], and selegiline [Eldepryl]). Other medicines that may also contribute to impaired thinking include those that treat bladder problems, high blood pressure, depression, anxiety, or insomnia.

In addition, standard tests may be done to evaluate memory problems, including a brain scan (CAT scan or MRI) and an EEG (electroencephalogram) or brain wave test. Common blood tests are also done, including thyroid studies, vitamin B_{12} levels, a screen for syphilis called an RPR or VDRL, as well as a routine blood count called a CBC and a chemistry panel to check for proper liver and kidney function. These tests are used to rule out other possible causes of dementia such as low thyroid levels, small strokes, and B_{12} deficiency. If a sudden change in behavior or thinking occurs, in addition to reviewing the medications, a physical exam and a screen for infection (of the urine or lungs) should be performed. You may also be referred to a psychologist for cognitive testing that involves several hours of pencil-and-paper questions to check your memory, verbal, and problem-solving skills.

If no specific cause is found for memory problems, some experts suggest incorporating daily activities to keep the mind and memory sharp. These activities can include hobbies or projects, crossword puzzles, exercise, and other interests.

When memory becomes less reliable, it becomes more important to make to-do lists and to keep a calendar and notepad with you at all times in order to jot down schedules, events, and things to remember. Some people prefer small electronic organizers or handheld computers.

Medications that have been proven to help in the dementia of Alzheimer's disease may also be very helpful in treating dementia found in persons with Parkinson's disease. These medicines—donepezil HCL (Aricept), rivastigmine tartrate (Excelon), and galantamine (Reminyl)—act by increasing the chemical acetylcholine in the brain and may improve memory and concentration.

If a person is having frequent hallucinations, and a complete physical examination and review and adjustment of medications fails to find a cause or relieve their presence, then treatment with atypical antipsychotic medicines such as quetiapine (Seroquel) or clozapine (Clozaril) should be considered.

Chapter 10

Special Issues for Patients and Caregivers

If you find it in your heart to care for somebody else, you will have succeeded.

—*Maya Angelou*

❖ YOUNG-ONSET PARKINSON'S DISEASE

Since popular actor Michael J. Fox announced that he has Parkinson's disease, the public and the medical community have become increasingly aware that younger people are not immune to this illness, and that even people in their thirties can be at risk. Fox's courage and advocacy in speaking out has forever dispelled the Parkinson's stereotype of the elderly person with a stooped posture, tremor, and slowed gait.

How common is Parkinson's disease in young people? Most Parkinson's disease specialists use the term *young-onset Parkinson's disease* (YOPD) when a patient develops symptoms before age 40. Approximately 5 to 10 percent of all persons with Parkinson's disease in North America and Europe have an onset before age 40. A very small percentage of YOPD patients are juvenile-onset Parkinson's disease or JP (juvenile Parkinson's), and develop symptoms before 21.

Pathologically, YOPD and adult-onset Parkinson's disease are the same, with the classic loss of dopamine neurons in the SNc (Substantia nigra compacta) and the presence of Lewy bodies. But YOPD differs from adult-onset Parkinson's disease in several ways. Younger patients tend to respond better to dopamine-stimulating drugs, and motor symptoms are more easily controlled. YOPD patients may also develop motor fluctuations such as "wearing off," "on-off," and dyskinesia earlier than adult-onset Parkinson's disease patients, sometimes within months or a year of starting levodopa therapy. It has been estimated that up to 55 percent of YOPD patients will develop dyskinesia within one year of starting levodopa, and 74 percent by the third year. This is much higher than the adult-onset rate of 28 to 50 percent experiencing dyskinesia and motor fluctuations 3 to 5 years after starting levodopa. Limb dystonia (sustained cramping and posturing of muscles) occurs early on in the course of Parkinson's disease in up to 43 percent of YOPD patients, compared to only 4 percent of adult-onset patients. Cognitive changes and difficulty with memory are far less common in YOPD. Young-onset patients do have motor symptoms of tremor, rigidity, and bradykinesia similar to older-onset Parkinson's disease patients but have less gait difficulty. It is generally agreed that YOPD progresses at a slower rate than adult-onset Parkinson's disease.

Getting Diagnosed

Getting an initial diagnosis of Parkinson's disease may be difficult for younger people—and it may even be delayed by many years—because some physicians aren't experienced in diagnosing YOPD.

Sam's story reflects this problem. Sam began noticing something was different around age 30.

> I felt shaky on the inside of my body and had difficulty holding my razor to shave. My hands felt stiff and achy. My family doctor prescribed an anti-inflammatory medication for arthritis. It didn't work and my symptoms got worse. A year later, after all the blood tests and X-ray reports failed to prove I had arthritis, I was referred to a neurologist, who diagnosed me with carpal tunnel syndrome. I wore wrist splints and took prescribed pain pills, but it didn't help. I knew something was wrong, but I didn't know what it was and neither did the doctors. Finally, I began to have bad tremors in both my hands and was referred to a different neurologist, who specialized in Parkinson's disease. She told me straight out that she thought I had Parkinson's disease. Even though I was only 33 years old, I was actually relieved to finally know what I had and to know that there was treatment available.

One patient, Joanne, had symptoms that started at the young age of 18, when she had trouble holding a pen at college.

> My body was stiff and sore and it was hard to get out of bed in the morning. My walking slowed down. I looked and felt like my grandmother. The doctors were baffled. My parents took me to so many different medical centers and I had so many blood tests and brain and body scans and even had to see several psychiatrists. Some of the doctors thought I was just de-

pressed, and having difficulty adjusting to college life. I was depressed, all right—depressed that no one but my parents believed me and no one could figure it out! Finally, after five years of searching, we found an expert doctor in Parkinson's disease and he knew right away that I had it. I was started on Sinemet and it was like a miracle, my body was free again to move. . . . The most important thing I can recommend to a young person with Parkinson's disease is to find a doctor who specializes in Parkinson's disease. It makes such a difference.

Treatments

YOPD should be treated differently than adult-onset Parkinson's disease, particularly with regard to medications. Because of the greater risk of developing motor fluctuations ("wearing off," "on-off," and dyskinesia) with levodopa in YOPD, levodopa therapy should be delayed for as long as possible, and dopamine agonists, amantadine, and anticholinergics considered for the treatment of disabling motor symptoms. Many patients will need to add levodopa within three to five years of beginning medication therapy to adequately control the tremors, bradykinesia, and rigidity. The goal at this time should be to use a combination of medications, such as a dopamine agonist with levodopa, in order to allow for a lower dose of levodopa, which reduces the risk of developing motor fluctuations.

Younger patients may find it difficult to accept that their bodies may at times be stiffer, slower, or shakier; they may want to be completely rid of all symptoms of Parkinson's disease, and will often request more medication to do so. But it is important to accept the presence of some Parkinson's disease motor symptoms that stem from taking less medication, in order to avoid some of the immediate and long-term side effects of taking more medication. YOPD patients also need to watch carefully for cognitive side effects from the medications, such as mental dulling or daytime sleepiness, as most young-onset patients are actively employed and need to remain particularly alert.

Another factor to consider in the treatment of YOPD persons is the possible need for surgical therapy. When a 32-year-old is diagnosed with Parkinson's disease, ten years later, at age 42, he or she still has a long life to lead, compared to a 75-year-old, who will likely have adequate control of the Parkinson's disease motor symptoms for the remainder of his or her life. If the YOPD person develops disabling motor fluctuations and if the motor symptoms are not as well controlled by the medications, surgical treatments can offer tremendous improvement in daily motor function and a return to independence.

Sherry was diagnosed with Parkinson's disease at age 38, and she has found that surgery was a tremendous help to her:

> After only eight years of having Parkinson's disease, I decided to have deep brain stimulation (DBS) surgery. I felt so helpless because I had horrible dyskinesia where my arms and legs would wiggle nonstop, sometimes all day. If I lowered the dose of my medicine, then I was so slow I couldn't even get up off the couch or walk or swallow. It's almost a year since my last surgery. I had an electrode put into the right side of my brain first and six months later I had another electrode put into the left side. It was the best decision I ever made. I am about 70 percent improved, with almost

no dyskinesia. I can do almost everything for myself again.

Coping with Young-Onset Parkinson's Disease

Being diagnosed with Parkinson's disease at a younger age can seem catastrophic. It is very common for a younger person to be in shock and often in denial after receiving such news. But it's important to be patient with yourself, and realize that Parkinson's disease is not a death sentence, nor the end of your world. You will survive, and you too will have your stories to share.

Alan remembers when he was diagnosed at age 38, 30 years ago:

> If I could have seen into the future to today, I would have felt a lot better when my doctor told me I had Parkinson's disease. I have had tremors and slowness and dyskinesia for a long time, but I can still walk and pretty much take care of myself; my wife helps me with buttoning and getting up out of bed before my medication kicks in. I have seen people who are much worse than me, and I think I am lucky. After thirty years of Parkinson's disease, I'm not afraid of it or what my future holds. I'm just glad to still be here.

Probably the most prominent young-onset Parkinson's disease patient in the United States, actor Michael J. Fox, was diagnosed with Parkinson's in 1991, at age 30. Fox, who has formed a foundation to search for a cure, has become a visible figure in the struggle for greater awareness of Parkinson's. But Fox's approach to coping with the condition is that he refuses to be defined by it. Instead he said he's been enhanced by it, describing himself as a "fuller person." Says Fox: "I'm living with it. And it is okay. I'm still me—me with Parkinson's."

Mary Noone, a Glenwood Springs, Colorado, artist whose Parkinson's disease appeared nine years ago, at age 37, feels that it is important for young-onset Parkinson's patients to be upfront about having the condition.

I tell everybody I have it, because it makes me uncomfortable to be shaking. People have even thought I was drinking, et cetera, so I think it's best to be very honest with your friends, family, and people you come into contact with. Ultimately, the more you get the information out there, the more chance there is that somebody is going to come back with an answer.

The impact on your career and family can also be a concern. There are so many questions a newly diagnosed YOPD patient is likely to ask: How long will I be able to work? Will I have to change the kind of work I do? What is my disability insurance? How will this affect my marriage, our retirement plan, the children's college? These are very valid and real concerns. Each person is different, with a different career or job, different stages and symptoms of Parkinson's, different financial and family resources, and different needs and goals. Learning how to adapt and change as life and health changes becomes an important skill.

Susie, a 48-year-old former pediatric intensive care unit nurse, was diagnosed with Parkinson's disease at age 32.

I did well for the first seven or eight years after being diagnosed with Parkinson's disease. I did have to take my medication on a strict schedule every four hours and often had to take an extra Sinemet pill while I was at work to get an extra boost so I could write and use my hands. I talked to my employer early on about Parkinson's disease, and they were wonderful and really worked with me; after four years I changed from a twelve-hour shift to an eight-hour one, which really helped. After eight years it became more difficult to keep up with the demands of ICU nursing; I was more fatigued and had more difficulty with writing and using needles, so I changed to nursing education part-time and am receiving partial medical disability. The best thing for me was to have a compassionate and understanding boss and coworkers.

Success Tips for YOPD Patients

- Talk about your illness with someone you trust early on. *Don't go it alone!*
- Consider seeing a professional counselor. Dealing with a serious illness at a young age can be extremely painful emotionally and psychologically, and your family may be struggling along beside you and not able to offer you the advice and understanding that you need.
- If you have children at home, have them access the Web site http://www.coles.org.uk/pdkids.htm. This is for children under age 18 who have parents or other family members with Parkinson's disease. They can talk to other kids in the same situation by joining a listserv. To join, send an e-mail to join-pd@lyris.parkinsons.org.uk.

- Find a young-age support group, and if one is not available, talk to other YOPD patients and try to start one; this can be an informal social gathering or an organized educational forum. Make it what you want and need it to be, and let it evolve over time. Discussing your particular needs, frustrations, and coping strategies regarding Parkinson's disease with other young patients can be an uplifting and freeing experience.
- Find a doctor who specializes in Parkinson's disease.
- Educate yourself (get a newsletter, buy a book, get online). Knowledge is power!
- Exercise, exercise, exercise!
- When you are ready, consider talking to your employer about your health to involve them in any possible changes in your duties at work and to plan for the future.
- If you are really struggling with performing your work duties, discuss this with your employer and your doctor to seek solutions with their help.
- Meet with a financial advisor and review your life, health, disability, and retirement plans.
- Consider marriage or couples counseling to help develop relationship strategies for coping with the disease.
- Do not be consumed by the diagnosis of Parkinson's disease. Review chapter 1 so that you truly understand that you are *not* your disease.

❖ JUST FOR CAREGIVERS

A caregiver is the person who routinely delivers care to the person with Parkinson's disease. Care can range from helping the person with Parkinson's disease do simple daily tasks such as getting out of bed, getting dressed, bathing, or going to a doctor's appointment, to reminding them to take medication on time, to spending time just listening or talking, and expressing one's love and concern for that individual.

A caregiver can be a bedside nurse, a dedicated spouse, an adult son or daughter, a grandchild, a sister or brother, a loyal friend, or a neighbor. If you know and help care for someone with Parkinson's disease on a regular basis—whether daily or weekly—then you are a caregiver. You can make the daily world of the person with Parkinson's manageable, livable, and very enjoyable. So if you are a caregiver, stand up right now and take a bow!

The topic of caregiving is a book all its own, as there's no possible way to cover all of the important issues that need to be discussed. But a few key points are covered here.

Essentials for Caregivers

First, be sure your own health will allow you to take on this role. Caregiving sometimes requires physical strength—such as helping a person with Parkinson's disease up from a fall or in and out of cars—and stamina. If you have serious health or physical limitations of your own, you may not be able to be the primary caregiver. Acknowledge this early on, so that you can seek other caregivers for you and the person you care for.

Another essential is patience. Parkinson's patients will often move slowly, and require extra time to accomplish what seem to be even the simplest tasks. Your patience will go a long way toward a successful caregiving relationship.

Also, understand that Parkinson's is not a static condition. What a person with Parkinson's disease can do may change, literally from hour to hour. It is critical that caregivers realize and recognize the variability and fluctuation of symptoms. Someone who was able to get up and walk comfortably in the morning may be barely able to move by afternoon. Caregivers might sometimes think this is a matter of will or even laziness—"If he tried harder he could get up by himself"—but these sorts of fluctuations are common. Learn to recognize the signs, so you and the person you care for can adapt to fluctuations.

Knowledge is essential. Find out as much as you can about Parkinson's disease, so you can understand and anticipate the condition of the person you care for and the challenges he or she faces. There are a variety of excellent resources that provide information and support to caregivers of people with Parkinson's disease. Organizations such as the National Parkinson Foundation, the American Parkinson's Disease Association, Parkinson's Disease Foundation, the Parkinson's Action Network, the Parkinson's Resource Organization, and the National Family Caregivers Association (NFCA) all offer support to the caregivers and families of Parkinson's patients and publish materials specifically for caregivers. The resources appendix lists many support groups, books, magazines, Web sites, videos, and other resources; all are excellent ways to find out more about Parkinson's disease.

Care for the Caregiver: Avoiding Burnout

A key issue is to make sure to take care of yourself and avoid burnout. Being a caregiver for someone who has Parkinson's disease can be very time-consuming, physically and emotionally demanding, and totally draining. Caregivers run the risk of becoming depleted of this energy or of becoming "burnt out." Here are some key ways to avoid burnout:

- Caregivers may want to attend a support group, in person or online.
- Make time for yourself every day (even twenty minutes of sitting quietly in your garden or reading a book or going for a walk can be invigorating).
- Encourage the person you care for to be as independent as they can be. Don't do everything!
- Ask the person you are caring for to do something for you, every day. It doesn't matter how small that thing is—it could be making the bed, helping with dinner, or rubbing your feet—but pick something that makes you happy that he or she can do for you.
- Get as many additional persons to help you in your role as caregiver (even one or two people to help can give you a well-deserved break and lighten your load).
- Pick at least one interest or hobby and pursue it weekly without the person you care for. This could be going to a movie, knitting, taking a cooking class, exercising, or any activity you enjoy.
- Get enough rest and sleep for yourself.

Cathie and John have been married for forty years, and John has had Parkinson's disease for the last fifteen of them. He has Stage IV Parkinson's disease and requires help with over 70 percent of his daily tasks. He struggles with walking, needing a cane or walker, and also has daily disabling dyskinesia. Cathie is a dedicated, loving spouse, and she spends much of her day helping John, but she also spends at least two to four hours of every day doing things for herself. She has several girlfriends she sees socially, plays bridge every Wednesday with the girls, goes to the grocery store, and takes a yoga class at the gym. She brings John along as much as possible in order to stimulate him. She has a neighbor who stays with John on the days she is away for longer periods, and her son helps to bathe him on the weekends. Says Cathie:

> We have a loving relationship that has changed as a result of Parkinson's, but still there is love and joy and understanding by both of us of each other's needs. We do as much as we can together, go out with friends or invite them over, rent or go to a movie, and attend the monthly Parkinson's disease support group. John understands that I do not have Parkinson's disease and I am not as slowed down and I want and need to see my friends and be more active than he can be. I am healthier and our relationship is better by me keeping some independence. I look forward to being with him after I have been out of the house. He usually has a friend over while I am gone, or is able to read or watch television to pass the time.

The Benefits and Rewards of Caregiving

Ruth Hagestuen, M.A., R.N., who serves as national program director for the National Parkinson Foundation, is concerned that we can endlessly discuss the challenges and strategies for the "doing" part of caregiving, while tending not to recognize the potential benefits and rewards of caregiving. Hagestuen feels that caregiving is potentially the most significant role each of us can undertake in our lifetime.

> The needs of family caregivers and the development of resources and systems to support those needs have been gravely underaddressed in our society. Lack of

preparation for the physical and emotional challenges is a health hazard. Chronic stress impacts the immune system and can lead to a variety of health problems. Statistics show indications of a health decline among spousal caregivers. These statistics can be changed and the experience of caregiving restored to be the experience where the rewards outweigh the trials and result in a healthy environment of care for both spouses.

Hagestuen notes that family caregivers report that the majority of their time is spent with housework, meals, laundry, groceries, and activities of daily living such as feeding and dressing. Basically, the majority finds their time is consumed in *doing*.

This leaves inadequate time for just *being* with oneself and one's carepartner . . . time for being in loving connection with each other . . . for being in the relationship. It is about having the opportunity to slow down long enough to appreciate and embrace the positive and the potentials. We need to find ways to maximize the good times to be had in caregiving. When my mother was severely compromised physically and verbally by a very complicated case of Parkinson's disease, we all would sit with her, telling and retelling stories of our childhood. These were very happy moments for her. She was very present as she listened, laughed, and cried with us. Ultimately, Parkinson's disease cannot take away the spirit or what the spirit allows one to see and hear: beautiful sunsets, the laughter of children, or the jokes of friends.

❖ FINDING AND EFFECTIVELY DEALING WITH DOCTORS

One of the most important issues a Parkinson's disease patient faces is finding and assembling the best team of practitioners, and then effectively communicating with them for optimal care and wellness.

Typically, for a Parkinson's disease patient, that team of practitioners would include your general practitioner and a neurologist. A good neurologist is essential. Neurologists specialize in treating disorders of the nervous system, including Parkinson's. In choosing a neurologist, someone who has expertise and interest in Parkinson's disease—also known as a movement disorder specialist—is likely to be informed on the latest findings regarding drug and surgical treatments for Parkinson's disease. If you are having surgery for Parkinson's, you'll want a surgeon who specializes in brain surgery—known as a neurosurgeon.

One way to find neurologists with a specific focus on Parkinson's patients is to go to a Parkinson's center. A number of reputable centers are recognized by the National Parkinson Foundation as Centers of Excellence. A list of these centers is featured in Appendix A.

You may also need to bring other experts onto your team. According to Eileen Savard, M.D., a patient advocate and author of *How to Save Your Own Life*:

> Parkinson's disease is a chronic illness that requires expertise and management by both a neurologist and a primary care practitioner. In fact, often patients require management by a number of specialists, including evaluations for urinary incontinence (urologist,

nurse specialists, et cetera), constipation (gastroenterologist or surgeon), seborrheic dermatitis (dermatologist), and physical therapist or rehab person, to
mention a few.

Holistic Practitioners

It's important for Parkinson's patients to have at least one holistically oriented practitioner on the team, because Parkinson's is
not always satisfactorily treated with purely conventional medicine. Ideally, a holistically oriented general practitioner or
neurologist would be optimal, because he or she can work with
you to safely and effectively integrate both conventional and
alternative therapies for your Parkinson's care. But a good holistic herbalist or nutritionist can also help you in integrating
alternatives into your treatment, and help you consider complementary approaches such as t'ai chi, Reiki, yoga, or even
herbal supplements.

There is a small but growing group of neurologists who are
integrating alternative and complementary approaches in their
practice. To find an alternative-minded neurologist, you'll
need to do some networking, ask around, talk to Parkinson's
support group members in your area, and ask holistic physicians for ideas and referrals. Some of the most innovative research is going on at the more than fifty designated National
Parkinson Foundation Centers of Excellence in the United
States, and doctors at these centers may be involved in alternative and complementary research.

Other options for holistic practitioners include:

* Osteopathic physicians—known as a "D.O.," or doctor of
  osteopathy—treat people holistically, and instead of treat-

ing each symptom separately, they look for the overall cause and attempt to treat the whole person.

- Holistic M.D.s tend to view patients as individuals, rather than as "members of a disease category," and incorporate patient autonomy and the use of the healing powers of love, hope, humor, and other positive forces into their treatment approaches.

- Orthomolecular physicians look at balancing the vitamins, minerals, and amino acids in the body, and use appropriate supplementation to achieve optimal nutritional balance and disease prevention and treatment.

- Doctors of oriental medicine typically use the accreditation D.O.M. or O.M.D. after their names. To find a qualified doctor of oriental medicine, and you live in a state that licenses such practitioners, seek a licensed practitioner. If you live in an area that does not regulate these practitioners, you should look for a practitioner who is board certified by the National Certification Commission for Acupuncture and Oriental Medicine (NCCAOM) or the American Association of Oriental Medicine.

- Herbalists are another option. Make sure you find a practitioner who has substantial experience, a good clientele, and a good reputation in the community, who has demonstrated clear knowledge, and is not simply trying to sell supplements. Members of the American Herbalists Guild, a prestigious membership organization for a select group of herbalists in the United States, are usually experienced enough to tackle complex conditions like Parkinson's disease.

Appendix A in this book lists organizations and Web sites that can help you find a neurologist, osteopath, holistic doctor, herbalist, and other specialists.

Finding a Great Doctor

Many times, finding the right neurologist, or even primary care doctor, is truly the best step toward getting better treatment—or even in getting diagnosed in the first place. To find a great doctor, there are a few key factors to consider:

- **Location and Affiliations**: Is the location of the doctor's office important to you? How far can you—or are you willing to—travel to see the doctor? Is it important to you that the doctor has privileges with or treats patients at a particular hospital?
- **Demographics**: Is the age, race, or religion of the doctor important to you? Will you feel more comfortable with a male or female doctor? Your gender preference may also be determined by what style you prefer. Research has found, for example, that women doctors typically spend more time with patients than do male colleagues.
- **Cost and Coverage**: You'll need to decide if you need a doctor who is part of your HMO or insurance program, because that financial decision is important to make at the onset, as it can focus your search. If you are restricted to plan-approved doctors from your HMO or health plan, ask the company whether they provide assistance in selecting doctors from their lists. Some may be able to provide profiles or more in-depth information about plan doctors.
- **Experience**: The level of experience you want will be determined by your personal preferences. Some younger doc-

tors may be more open to or knowledgeable about alternative medicine, or less imperious. Older doctors, however, might seem more reassuring, with greater expertise and better bedside manner. Your choice really depends on your own preferences.

- **Certification**: Particularly with neurologists, you'll want a board-certified neurologist. Board-certified neurologists are members of the American Board of Psychiatry and Neurology.
- **Record**: You may want to check that there are no disciplinary actions filed against a particular doctor. One key place to find out: Public Citizen's *Questionable Doctors* listings, at http://www.citizen.org, or call 202-588-1000.
- **Availability/Flexibility**: Some people want a doctor who has evening or weekend hours, or who can see patients on short notice, or who will do consultations by phone.

Appendix A has a number of helpful organizations, including referral services and Web sites that can help you find potential doctors.

Karen tells of her experience looking for the right doctor:

My family doctor sent me to a local neurologist who diagnosed me with Parkinson's disease. That neurologist didn't tell me much about Parkinson's disease at all, just gave me a prescription and said come back in six months. Ultimately, I found a Parkinson center about two hours away. The first visit, the doctor spent an hour with me, not just examining my body, but talking to me about Parkinson's and what might cause it and the many treatments, including the need to adopt a healthier lifestyle, to exercise and lose weight, to take vitamins, to go to a support group, to read more and learn more about the medicine I was taking. This doctor listened to me and answered my questions and was very positive about me and maintaining my independence. The thing I learned the most from this experience is that it is worth taking the time and effort and even traveling a bit to find the right doctor. Don't settle for less than you want and deserve.

One you've narrowed down your selections and have a list of possible doctors, it's time to conduct a brief screening interview by phone. During your call with the doctor and staff, some of the possible questions you might want to ask should include the following:

- Are you accepting new patients at this time?
- Is a physician referral required?
- Are you an individual or group practice?
- If I have an appointment with you, will I be seen by you or by another doctor?
- If I'm going to see another doctor, will I have advance notice?
- Who covers for you when you're unavailable?
- How long in advance do I have to make an appointment?
- Do you keep slots open for emergency appointments?
- Do you charge a fee for missed appointments? How much is it?
- Do you accept patient phone calls?
- Are calls scheduled for a specific time of day?
- How soon do you typically return calls?
- Do your nurses return calls for you?
- Is advice given over the phone?

- Do you accept patient e-mails?
- Do you accept patient faxes?
- What are your customary fees?
- Do you accept my health insurance coverage or Medicare?
- Is full payment (or deductibles or copayments) required at the time of the appointment?
- Are lab work and X-rays performed in the office?
- What hours are you available?
- Do you refer patients to alternative treatments?
- Can you provide several patient references I can speak with?

If a doctor's office isn't interested in providing you with at least some of this information in advance, then you may want to move on to someone else who is more responsive. Doctors who don't recognize that patients are clients to whom they provide a service often aren't productive in the long run.

Evaluating Your Relationship

Whether you're trying out a new doctor, or you've been with a particular doctor for a while, it's important to evaluate the relationship with the doctor. To help in that process, you can ask yourself these questions:

- Is your doctor patient and willing to explain the rationale for tests and treatments? Does he or she share options with you and allow you to participate in decision making?
- Is your doctor interested in partnering with you and helping to educate you, rather than just issuing orders, expecting you to follow them?

- Does your doctor believe in, work with, or encourage alternative, holistic, or complementary approaches?
- Does your doctor take time to get to know anything about you and your feelings? Does he or she truly listen?
- Does your doctor answer your questions, and not rush through your visits without covering your key concerns, and not become impatient when you ask for further explanations?
- Does your doctor and his or her office staff treat patients and others with courtesy and respect, not keep you waiting excessively, and return calls or faxes within a reasonable amount of time?
- Will your doctor read materials you provide to him or her?
- Does your doctor encourage you to do your own research?

For one Parkinson's patient, Randy, finding a doctor to help him with his Parkinson's was a challenge that involved visiting four different doctors over a three-year period of time before he was even diagnosed. Even then, the doctor who diagnosed his condition was, according to Randy, "a very old-fashioned and pessimistic 'super' Parkinson's disease specialist and chairman of a university neurology department. He was extremely negative in terms of the possibility of successful intervention, and he scared the heck out of my wife and me."

Randy's symptoms eventually reached a point where he and his wife feared that he would become significantly impaired, lose his mobility, and require constant assistance. Randy kept up the search, and he finally found a new doctor who better matched his needs.

> Her expertise and willingness to try numerous medications in attempting to help me resulted in an almost

miraculous reduction in my daily symptoms after seven years of diagnosis and treatment. After so many attempted medications and combinations, when I had all but given up, she tried again with amantadine. Within two weeks I was like 70 percent of my old self, walking upright with renewed balance, strength, and energy. Other changes followed, including hope and appreciation of so many small blessings that I took for granted before Parkinson's disease.

Randy's advice to any other Parkinson's disease patient is to persist until you "find the doctor that listens and hears you. But most of all the doctor you want is one who cares about patients and has a belief that there is treatment to help you."

The Empowered Patient's Records

According to Marie Savard, M.D., a patient advocate and author of *How to Save Your Own Life* and *The Savard Health Record*, everyone—and in particular patients with chronic illnesses such as Parkinson's disease—should keep a complete and organized medical file of their own. Says Dr. Savard:

The file should include sections for all medications ever prescribed, reactions to medicines, side effects experienced, allergies, specialist consultations, lab tests, preventive health information (such as vaccines received, cancer screenings), a chronological journal or section for each doctor visit, including findings and recommendations, hospital summaries, and operative reports. Each practitioner can add necessary information to this file, and patients should take their file to every doctor visit, so that every practitioner that needs to can take a look.

Dr. Savard has found that not only is maintaining this information important—perhaps even essential for health—but it also has a positive impact on attitude. According to Dr. Savard:

> Patients with Parkinson's disease feel they are losing control over their bodies, but having a copy of all their medical information makes them feel in control of the disease. What a gift! I can't tell you how powerful and secure people feel when they know each doctor they see has all their information at their fingertips.

There are a variety of ways you can keep track of this information. Some people keep a portable expandable accordion file. Others prefer a binder. Some prefer to type notes into a computer and to scan forms and records. Dr. Savard has also created an easy-to-use binder with pre-made tabs and forms, *The Savard Health Record*, that helps you organize and manage your medical information and visits.

A critical part of your medical information file should include information about the drugs and medications you use. Many people, and in particular Parkinson's patients, take a variety of different medicines. Since some medicines can have troublesome—even dangerous—side effects, it's important that your doctors be aware of all the medicines you take. In addition to prescription medications, this includes over-the-counter nonprescription drugs, such as vitamins, herbs, laxatives—even eye drops. Your personal health record should, for each drug, indicate how much of it you take, and how often you take it.

The Effective Appointment

An effective appointment with your doctor is in part your responsibility, and there are some techniques you can use to help make that appointment as productive as possible.

FILL OUT FORMS BEFORE YOUR FIRST VISIT

Request that the new doctor's office mail or fax you all their medical and information forms in advance of your visit, and fill them out ahead of time. This can be particularly helpful for Parkinson's patients who have difficulty writing legibly or who write slowly.

BRING ALONG A HEALTH BUDDY

It's rare that any one doctor is running the show for a chronically ill patient. It is critical, therefore, that a patient has a point person—what Dr. Savard calls a "health buddy"—to act as a central coordinator and advocate. Most often, that person is a spouse, family member, friend, or caregiver. The health buddy can help fill out medical forms at the doctor's office, plan the appointment agenda, remind you of what you planned to discuss with the doctor during the appointment, and even take notes or record what the doctor said during an appointment. And even if your health buddy can't go to an appointment, he or she can still help by being a sounding board, rehearsing key points you want to bring up with the doctor, or brainstorming with you to prioritize your questions for the doctor.

CREATE A WRITTEN AGENDA FOR APPOINTMENTS

A written agenda for your appointment can be a wonderful tool for a more effective session with your physician. Your agenda should include a list of your concerns, prioritized so that the most important items to be discussed are at the top of the list. Are you having new symptoms you want to discuss? Did you notice any side effects from your medicine? Did you want to get a flu shot? Put it down on the agenda. Your agenda should also include any important updates since your last visit. For example, if you were treated at the emergency room, or if you've had any changes in appetite, weight, or sleep habits, these are important to mention. If you've had any major life stresses it's also essential to mention this to your doctor. And be sure to bring extra copies for your doctor and health buddy, so everyone can review the agenda.

COMMUNICATE EFFECTIVELY

There are some important ways you can facilitate effective communications at your appointment. First, be honest with your doctor. Don't tell the doctor what you think he/she wants to hear; tell the truth. That's particularly important when it comes to side effects, smoking, exercise, diet, and other important issues. Next, ask questions. Otherwise, the doctor will assume you understand exactly what he or she is saying, and you don't need or want further information or explanation. Also, it's important to be direct. If you feel rushed, worried, or uncomfortable, be sure to speak up to try to get the doctor to focus on your concerns. For example, you may want to say "I know you have a busy schedule, but I'm very concerned about this. I'd feel better if we could talk about it a bit more." If a doctor simply can't spend any further time, ask when the doctor can schedule time to call you, or schedule a return visit if needed. You should also be careful not to forget to discuss your specific symptoms. This is where a health journal or health record can be of particular help, because you can keep track of when certain symptoms started, what time of day they occur, how long they typically last, when they occur and how often, and what seems to help or worsen the symptoms. Also, learn how to discuss sensitive subjects. Even if you are embarrassed or uncomfortable, it's important to raise subjects such as poor memory, depression, sexual function, and incontinence with your physician. Don't assume they are untreatable aspects of Parkinson's disease.

CAPTURE INFORMATION

Capturing information is particularly important. You and your doctor or practitioner will only have a short time together, and in the rush of the visit and covering your points, you may find it difficult to remember exactly what the doctor has said. One technique is to take notes. When it comes to complicated terms, or names of medications, you may even ask the doctor to write down the name for you. If you can't write while the doctor is talking to you, you may want to sit in the waiting room after the visit to record your notes while they are fresh in your mind. Taking notes is also a helpful role that your health buddy may perform on your behalf. Some patients like to bring a tape recorder along, and, with the doctor's permission, make a recording of the visit. Many doctors can also provide fact sheets, brochures, pamphlets, audiotapes, or videotapes that discuss conditions, drugs, and treatments. Ask your physician if he or she has educational information available to take home.

DEAL WITH DISSATISFACTION

When you have a misunderstanding with your physician, or with his or her staff, it's important to address it directly. Don't avoid the doctor—face the problem head-on. For example, if the doctor was not returning your telephone calls, you may want to say at your next appointment, "I understand that you have a heavy workload and are very busy, but I feel frustrated when I have to wait for days for you to return my call. How can we work together to resolve this?" If you need a fast response to a question, and you aren't successful in leaving a phone message, write up your concerns and fax them to your doctor's office. Faxes tend to get a quicker response than phone messages. (If you don't have a home fax, many copy centers will send a fax inexpensively.) And if problems are not resolvable, it's important to put your concerns in writing to the doctor and send a copy to your health insurance company, health maintenance organization's customer affairs department, your state health department, and the American Medical Association.

Note from Dr. Jill: Words Are the Most Powerful Medicine of All

We would all be wiser if we would listen more carefully to the words we say and take a little more time to choose them before saying them. But I particularly believe that physicians and health care professionals need to realize that the words they say may very well be more helpful or harmful to patients than the prescriptions they write or the treatments they administer.

Daniel was a patient of mine I had been treating for Parkinson's for about a year. He had very early, mild, unilateral Parkinson's disease. He was involved in a study for a new Parkinson's drug, and it was very hard to tell he even had Parkinson's when he took his medicine. To look at him, one would have thought he was doing well, but he was not. He was physically well, but emotionally he had been struggling with the acceptance of having been diagnosed with Parkinson's and had many fears about it.

During one visit, out of the blue he asked me, "Do you think I should buy a boat?"

"Do you want to buy a boat?" I asked.

"Oh yes," he said. "Now that I'm retired I've just been waiting to get my boat and go bass fishing."

So then I asked him if he had enough money to buy it, and he did, so I enthusiastically told him to go buy it and bring me back some pictures of the bass he caught—or, better yet, take me with him sometime. He got a big smile on his face. "Great, I already have it picked out. I'm going to go buy it this afternoon."

What he was really asking me was "Can I still fish even though I have Parkinson's?" He was afraid that he wouldn't live long enough to enjoy his boat and bass fishing. What if I hadn't really listened? What if I had said something ambivalent like "I guess so" or "I don't know" or "Maybe"? Or worse, what if I had said "I don't think you should buy it"? It may seem like this was an insignificant conversation to some people, but I don't believe it was. I believe that by the words I said and by how I said them, I told Daniel he would live a long while in spite of having been diagnosed with Parkinson's disease and that he should enjoy his retirement. I believe Daniel left that day a happier, more positive person.

Just as positive, caring words can have a dramatic impact upon patients by giving them hope, encouragement, or guidance, negative, unfeeling, or carelessly chosen words can do just the opposite, by taking away hope and creating unwanted fears, anxiety, or depression. One of my patients told me that the first doctor she saw who diagnosed her with Parkinson's disease said, "Do you think you know more than me about Parkinson's disease? You just let me tell you what to do, I'm the doctor here." Needless to say, she never went back to see him again.

We are all guilty, myself included, of saying things we regret, or simply not thinking before we open our mouths, and not realizing the impact of the words we are about to say. In the world of medicine, we have to do a better job; we have the power to hurt or help with the words we say.

And so if you are a person with Parkinson's, I strongly encourage you to seek out health professionals who talk to you on your level, listen, and are positive in their behavior—especially in the words they use. I also encourage you to let them know if they have said something that has upset you. Dialogue should be a two-way street, and you should always voice your opinion loud and clear. Good, effective communication will allow you and your health care partners to provide better treatment for you.

Part V

PARKINSON'S INTO THE FUTURE

Chapter 11

Future Directions

We must accept finite disappointment, but never lose infinite hope.

—*Martin Luther King, Jr.*

Although there are good, effective treatments for Parkinson's disease currently available, it is clear that we still have a long way to go in finding more effective treatments—whether via drugs, surgery, or greater understanding of what causes Parkinson's disease—so that we can look at potential preventative or curative therapies for the future.

In the drug arena, new medications to treat the motor and nonmotor symptoms of Parkinson's disease need to be found. Neuroprotective agents to preserve brain cells need to be developed. Better long-term study of the surgical treatments of Parkinson's disease needs to occur, so that we can better understand the long-term benefits and possible complications. Alternative therapies need to be studied, to validate their use in the treatment of Parkinson's disease.

In the area of genetics, identification of new genes linked to the cause of Parkinson's disease, as well as epidemiological studies to find possible environmental factors, must be carried out. Neurostem cells and other potential tissue transplants need to be studied further.

The exciting news is, all of this is happening now. All of these areas are being studied now. And it's clear that our knowledge of the causes and triggers of Parkinson's disease, and better treatments for the condition, will continue to grow and flourish. The future is bright and full of hope and promise.

❖ NEW THEORIES ABOUT THE CAUSE OF PARKINSON'S DISEASE

When the cause of a disease is unknown, as in the case of Parkinson's disease, many theories are formulated by experts to explain the possible causes. These theories are extremely important, as future research will depend on these theories. Some of the most cutting-edge theories about what causes dopamine cell death in Parkinson's disease include the following:

- Oxidative stress and free radicals
- Mitochondrial defect in complex I
- Excitotoxicity
- Inflammation
- Apoptosis
- Protein clumping

Oxidative Stress, Free Radicals, and Mitochondrial Defects

The theory that oxidative stress and free radicals, and mitochondrial impairment in complex I, both can lead to dopamine cell death has been introduced in chapter 1. To briefly review, a buildup of free radicals in the brain could lead to dopamine cell death and impaired complex I activity in the mitochondria, the energy producer of each living cell. When cells are impaired, this can easily result in the inability of the dopamine cell to produce the necessary energy to survive.

The importance of these theories, which are intimately linked to one another, is that many targeted therapies and current research are aimed at decreasing free-radical formation through the use of antioxidants, which bind free radicals to prevent damage to the cell.

Excitotoxicity

Excitotoxicity refers to the idea that excessive stimulation of the brain by the excitatory chemical glutamate may lead to dopamine cell death. Excitotoxicity has long been proven to be a cause of damage to brain cells. Glutamate binds to three main glutamate receptors—NMDA, AMPA, and kainate—and glutamate directly binds to these receptors. Some of the new drugs for Parkinson's disease are targeted at blocking glutamate receptors. When glutamate receptors are activated or "excited" by glutamate, an increase flow of calcium into the cell may occur. This increased calcium flow can activate certain cell enzymes—proteases, lipases, and endonucleases—that break down important cell proteins. This breakdown of proteins may cause serious injury or death of the brain cell.

A high concentration of glutamate occurs in the brain, especially in the subthalamic nucleus (STN), which connects to the substantia nigra compacta (SNc) dopamine brain cells. These dopamine cells—the ones that are affected in Parkinson's disease—have a large number of glutamate receptors. It has been shown that rats and primates given the Parkinson-inducing drug MPTP are protected against dopamine cell death when they are given an NMDA receptor antagonist that blocks glutamate activity. This supports the concept that blocking glutamate may protect dopamine cells from toxic damage.

Future research will focus on looking at more effective drugs or treatments that would block glutamate receptors and protect dopamine cells.

Inflammation

Inflammation as a theory for dopamine cell death is not as widely accepted, but deserves consideration and further evaluation. The body and brain have natural immune system responses that are triggered in response to an infection, toxins, or some other type of cell injury. These immune responses involve a variety of inflammatory cells and molecules, the most important of these in the brain being the microglia and cytokines. Large numbers of reactive microglia have been shown to exist in the substantia nigra compacta (SNc) in persons with Parkinson's disease on postmortem examination. The cytokines that microglia produce can trigger a cascade of inflammatory reactions and subsequent neuronal cell death. They act as a kind of garbage disposal by cleaning up and getting rid of debris in response to cell injury. Higher amounts of the cytokines interleukin 1 and 6 have been reported in the cerebrospinal fluid of persons with Parkinson's disease.

In addition, glutathione is made by the microglia and is delivered to neurons in response to excitatory stimulation. Low levels or loss of glutathione occurs early in Parkinson's disease, implicating the microglia. Whether the microglia and some of the cytokines and other neurotoxic molecules they produce can be activated and cause dopamine cell death remains open to debate. It may be that their involvement is simply a by-product of dopamine cell injury and a normal response to this. Whether anti-inflammatory agents for the treatment of Parkinson's disease will be effective also remains to be seen.

Research is already under way into the use of glutathione supplementation as a protective agent, and other anti-inflammatory therapies will undoubtedly be the subject of future research.

Apoptosis

Apoptosis is defined as gradual, slow, programmed cell death. The cell that undergoes apoptosis shrinks in size, has no inflammatory reaction, has a preserved cell membrane, and undergoes breakdown of the DNA. This is very different from necrosis of a cell, which is much faster and involves the influx of calcium and breakdown of cell proteins, disruption of the mitochondrial energy production, and cell membrane rupture and secondary inflammation. Many of the cells in the brain and spinal cord of developing embryos, before and soon after birth, undergo apoptosis or programmed cell death. This ensures that the correct number and type of cells are made. This type of apoptosis is controlled by formation of specific proteins, and inhibiting the formation of these proteins can block the programmed apoptosis. The proteins that are necessary for apoptosis are always present in some cells and have to be manufactured in other cells.

A number of agents that are implicated in playing a role in the cause of dopamine cell death in Parkinson's disease have been shown to cause apoptosis, including glutathione deficiency, the synthetic drugs MPTP and MPP+, 6-hydroxydopamine, high iron levels, mitochondrial complex I inhibitors, and excitatory agents. Studies have shown that low levels of the toxin MPP+ caused apoptosis in laboratory embryonic dopamine cells, while higher concentrations caused necrosis. Medium concentrations caused both necrosis and apoptosis. It also appears that apoptosis involves the mitochondria, in that one of the proteins found in the mitochondria, cytochrome C, can trigger apoptosis if released into the cells' fluid.

Where these developments most impact the future of Parkinson's disease is that the genes that regulate apoptosis have actually been discovered. The gene for superoxide dismutase (SOD), a free-radical scavenger, for example, decreases apoptosis when it is "turned on" and increases apoptosis when it is "turned off." These are extremely important findings, because future drugs may be able to target those specific genes and halt or slow apoptosis of dopamine cells or other brain cells. These types of drugs could then help to slow or even prevent Parkinson's and other similar diseases such as Alzheimer's disease.

Protein Clumping

Protein clumping, or aggregation, has been reported to occur in the dopamine cell and is thought to result in the formation of the Lewy body and possibly in disruption of cellular function and subsequent cell death. Much of the recent reports of protein aggregation are born out of genetic studies of familial forms of Parkinson's disease. One of the most important findings in the last five years has been the identification of a mutation in a gene on chromosome number 4 that is thought to cause the development of Parkinson's disease in people who have inherited this gene. A small change in the gene (which leads to a single amino acid substitution) results in malformation of the protein alpha-synuclein. This protein is found within and makes up the core of the Lewy body in both familial (inherited) and sporadic (unknown cause) Parkinson's disease. Normally, alpha-synuclein helps maintain the cell membrane (the walls of the cell) and neurotransmitter vesicle function (the pouches that contain the cell's chemicals, e.g., dopamine). It is thought that unhealthy or mutant alpha-synuclein may disrupt the normal cell membrane and neurotransmitter activity. The neurotransmitter vescicles needs to remain healthy so as to allow proper packaging and transport of dopamine. This is important to preserve cell function and survival and prevent cellular death of dopamine neurons.

Another key protein found in the Lewy body is ubiquitin. When proteins are old or damaged, they need to be broken down and removed for the cell to remain healthy. Ubiquitin does this by binding to damaged or misfolded proteins and presenting them to proteasomes. The proteasomes then break down the protein into smaller pieces that can be used to make new proteins for the cell. Parkin, another protein that functions in a similar manner as ubiquitin, may malfunction due to a gene mutation on chromosome number 6 in very-young-age-onset parkinsonism.

If ubiquitin malfunctions or becomes overwhelmed, then proteins will build up into clumps, called protein aggregates. These and similar protein aggregates have been found in Parkinson's disease brain cells, as well as in other neurodegenerative diseases such as Alzheimer's and Huntington's disease. It is possible that protein clumping may lead to cell death, similar to a garbage disposal that stops working because it is clogged with too much garbage or debris.

❖ THE DEVELOPMENT OF NEW DRUGS

It is important to have some understanding of how new medications are studied before they become available and can be prescribed by your physician. Once a company has developed a new drug, the drug must go through a very lengthy process of specific studies, typically lasting anywhere from ten to fifteen years or more. Most drugs are first studied in animal models of the disease to check for toxicity and clinical benefit.

For testing of Parkinson's disease drugs, the most common models used are the 6-hydroxydopamine (6-OHDA) rat model and the MPTP rat and monkey models. These toxic agents (6-OHDA and MPTP), when delivered to the brain of a rat or monkey, cause a loss of dopamine cells in the brain of the animal and a clinical appearance similar to Parkinson's disease, with tremors, rigidity, and slowness of movement.

Once animal studies have been completed, if the drug appears to be safe and potentially helpful, then human studies begin. Each drug must then pass through a series of phased studies.

- **Phase I** involves testing a new drug or treatment in a small group of subjects (twenty to eighty people) for the first time to look for side effects, judge the safety of the drug, and determine safe dosage ranges. These studies typically involve healthy volunteers.

- **Phase II** involves testing a new drug or treatment on a larger group of people (one hundred to three hundred subjects) who have the target symptoms or illness (e.g., Parkinson's disease) that the drug is intended to help. Phase II judges how effective the drug is and further evaluates for side effects and safety.

- **Phase III** involves testing a new drug or treatment on a much larger group of people (one thousand to three thousand subjects) to confirm its effectiveness (e.g., that it helps to reduce the motor symptoms of Parkinson's disease or to slow down the progression of Parkinson's disease or to lessen dyskinesia or wearing off), to monitor closely for side effects, compare it to other similar approved treatments, and collect information to be sure the drug or treatment can be used safely. After Phase III, a drug can be submitted to the Food and Drug Administration (FDA) for approval.

- **Phase IV** involves testing a new drug or treatment that has already passed through Phases I, II, and III and has been FDA-approved for prescription use. These studies may test for additional clinical benefits or look for a different clinical benefit that was not studied previously, as well as monitor for long-term safety.

As noted, once a drug has passed Phase III clinical trials, it can be submitted to the FDA for approval for use in patient treatment. If the drug is FDA-approved, a process that can take many months or even years, then it can be prescribed by a licensed physician or physician's assistant. All of the available medications for the treatment of Parkinson's disease discussed in chapter 5 had to complete this process. Overall, this process of animal testing, human clinical trials, and FDA review and approval strives to ensure the safety and effectiveness of a new drug.

◈ CLINICAL STUDIES: CAN YOU BELIEVE THEM?

"New Drug May Slow Parkinson's!" "Drug Offers Promise for Parkinson's Patients!" You may see or hear these sorts of headlines regularly reported in your newspapers, television news health segments, radio reports, or magazines. If you have access to medical journals or the Internet, you may also come upon journal articles or research abstracts that highlight new developments.

But remember that in order to be able to critically judge the validity of the study and its conclusions, you need to know where and how a study was performed, what type of study it was, who performed it, and how the results were interpreted. If you are a person without much scientific background, you might consider this to be an impossible task, but there are useful guidelines that can help you understand the definitions and terminology used in clinical studies.

First, when reading or hearing of any results or reports of new treatments for Parkinson's disease, be sure to find out the exact source. Whether this was a national or local news report, a radio report, a verbal report by a doctor or friend, or from the Internet, you should get the exact reference. That means finding out whether the study was published, and if so, in what journal. Ideally, you should get a copy of the original report and review it with your physicians and health care professionals. Breakthrough treatments are rare, but if they are true, they should be published in reputable, peer-reviewed medical or basic science journal.

Once you have the study in hand, some questions you and your practitioner should consider include the following:

- What is the exact source of the information? Is it a medical journal article, a summary of findings from a medical group meeting, an independent researcher, or other source?
- Is it a medically reputable source?
- What kind of study is it?
- How many persons participated in the study and for how long?
- Was it a placebo-controlled study? The term *placebo effect* refers to the bias that occurs when a person—patient or researcher—knows ahead of time the treatment that will be given; the belief that it will be helpful may cause the person to subconsciously report the results he or she expects to occur. In a placebo-controlled study of a new drug, for example, the patient may get the real new study drug or the fake drug, known as a placebo. To remove the placebo effect and any bias, both the researcher and study subject should be blinded if possible.
- Was it a single-blind placebo-controlled study? This means either the patient who is participating in the study or the person who evaluates the patient does not know what treatment is being given.
- Was it a double-blind placebo-controlled study? This means both the patient participating in the study and the researcher evaluating the patient do not know what treatment the person is receiving. Double-blinded studies are thought to be the most valid, because they remove any chance of patient and evaluator bias or placebo effect.
- Is the statistical analysis valid?
- What are the conclusions, and do they seem to reflect the study results reported?

- Are there other similar studies that conclude the same thing or contradict these results?
- Should I change my treatment for Parkinson's disease based on this study?
- If a new treatment for Parkinson's disease is being recommended, are there potential side effects or dangers involved that I should be aware of?
- If a new treatment is reported to be beneficial for the treatment of Parkinson's disease, is it readily available for use now or is it still in the study phase and yet to be approved by the FDA?

If you can begin to answer some of these questions with the help of your health care team, you will be able to know how to interpret what you have read or heard and how to use this information wisely.

It's common for patients to hear a national news report about some promising new findings recently published in some medical journal. They rush to the doctor, wanting to try it. But what the reporters failed to include in their report is that the treatment may not be available for general use and is currently only in clinical trials, or the study was performed on animal models and has yet to be even studied in human beings—meaning that practical treatments for patients are years away.

A good example of this is in the current national discussion of neurostem cells—known as stem cells—which is also mentioned later in this chapter. Some people with Parkinson's disease have the idea that neurostem cell transplants will be available very soon, and that they will cure their Parkinson's disease. Neurostem research is in its infancy, and has great potential for Parkinson's disease, but many years of research must take place before it can even be considered as a viable therapy for Parkinson's disease.

❖ NEW MEDICINES FOR SYMPTOMATIC TREATMENT OF PARKINSON'S DISEASE

There are a variety of new medications that are currently being studied for the treatment of the motor symptoms of Parkinson's disease. The goal is to find potent medications similar to levodopa that have less harmful side effects and that are more effective over longer periods of time.

Sumanirole

Dopamine agonists similar to the four available medications are being developed. One such drug is sumanirole, which in 2002 entered Phase III studies in patients with Parkinson's disease. The hope is that because it has a longer duration of action (perhaps allowing for twice-daily dosing rather than three-times-daily dosing), it may help prevent wearing off and may be associated with a lower risk of developing dyskinesia.

The Dopamine Patch

The dopamine patch has completed Phase II studies, and Phase III studies began in 2002. This is a unique drug that delivers a dopamine agonist transdermally, through the skin— much like the nicotine or estrogen patch. The patient places the patch on the skin of the shoulder or back and then takes it off twenty-four hours later and applies a new patch. This allows for more continuous delivery of medication and may thereby allow for a lower occurrence of "off" time or wearing off, and possibly lessen the risk of developing dyskinesia. If the person's symptoms were well controlled with the patch, then he or she might not even need to take any oral medication or be able to take less oral pills during the day. This could be a great relief to the many patients who take medicine as frequently as every one to three hours.

The common side effects that have occurred with the dopamine patch are nausea, vomiting, sedation, and confusion. Some patients experienced a rash where the patch was applied. If a person does experience side effects, they may last longer, as the medication is continuously being absorbed and delivered to the bloodstream and brain. This could be a drawback, when the patch is compared to oral medication.

An abstract report on Rotigotine Transdermal System (SMP-962) from the Fourteenth International Congress on Parkinson's Disease (2001) stated it to be an effective and beneficial drug for the treatment of Parkinson's disease. The study enrolled 242 Parkinson's disease patients who were randomized to wear a placebo patch or the dopamine patch, which they used for twelve weeks. Those using the actual dopamine patch had a significant improvement in their motor rating scales, compared to those who used the placebo patch. It is anticipated that after completion of Phase III trials, the dopamine patch will be available for prescription use, pending FDA approval.

❖ TREATMENT OF NONMOTOR SYMPTOMS AND SIDE EFFECTS

In addition to the medications that treat the motor symptoms of Parkinson's disease, some medications currently under development may help treat some of the side effects that result from Parkinson's disease medicines, or help treat some of the nonmotor symptoms of Parkinson's disease.

For example, aripiprazole, a new antipsychotic drug, is being studied for the treatment of schizophrenia and might also be studied in the future for the treatment of hallucinations in patients with Parkinson's disease. The hope is that it would lessen hallucinations caused as a side effect from Parkinson's disease drugs without worsening the motor symptoms.

New breakthroughs for the treatment of Alzheimer's dementia might also help Parkinson's disease persons with disabling dementia. Safer and more effective drugs for the treatment of urinary frequency or incontinence, impotence, low blood pressure, depression, dementia, sedation, and insomnia could be very helpful for the patient who has any of these symptoms.

New medicines to lessen the risk of developing dyskinesia are now being developed. One such drug is idazoxan. This is an alpha-2-adrenoreceptor antagonist, which blocks noradrenaline. The researchers theorize that noradrenaline—which is made from levodopa—may cause dyskinesia, and that by blocking the formation or activity of noradrenaline, the degree of dyskinesia will lessen. One study showed that marmosets treated with idazoxan had a 75 percent reduction in dyskinesia using a blinded rater. A small study of eighteen people with Parkinson's disease, published in the same journal, showed some reduction in dyskinesia compared to placebo. Similar alpha-adenosine receptor blockers were to begin Phase II and Phase III human studies in 2002 and 2003 for the reduction of dyskinesia.

Another class of drugs, called 5-HT1A agonists, which includes the drug sarizotan, has been shown in animal models of Parkinson's disease to reduce levodopa-induced dyskinesia by as much as 91 percent. This drug will likely be studied in human Parkinson's disease trials.

◈ NEUROPROTECTIVE AGENTS

A neuroprotective agent is something that protects the nervous system; in the case of Parkinson's disease, this means protection of the dopamine brain cell by preventing it from injury and subsequent death. A neuroprotective agent could arrest or slow down the rate of progression of Parkinson's disease such that a person diagnosed at 40 with Parkinson's disease might be able to maintain independent motor function for more than twenty years with such a drug. Currently, we do not have a proven neuroprotective agent for Parkinson's disease, but many such drugs are being studied and developed today. The discovery of an effective neuroprotective drug could be the next major breakthrough for the treatment of Parkinson's disease, and many Parkinson's specialists believe that this could occur within the next decade.

Selegiline (Eldepryl, Deprenyl)

Selegiline—also known as Eldepryl and Deprenyl—was the first drug touted as a possible neuroprotective agent. This came about because of the observation that selegiline blocks the conversion of MPTP to MPP+, which is a potent toxin to dopamine cells. It has not, however, been proven to slow the progression of Parkinson's disease, but rather allows levodopa to remain in its original form and to work longer at controlling the motor symptoms of Parkinson's disease. Selegiline was shown to protect dopamine neurons in the MPTP animal models of Parkinson's disease because it stops the conversion of

MPTP to the neurotoxin MPP+. Even though selegiline has not been fully accepted as a neuroprotective agent, it is possible that one of its breakdown products, desmethylselegiline, may be one. Desmethylselegiline appears to protect brain cells from excitotoxicity and glutathione depletion and may do so by increasing the brain's natural levels of growth factors, which may help nourish brain cells and protect them from premature cell death. This has been recently reported to occur in mice that were given desmethylselegiline. Because selegiline and other related drugs have the potential to be neuroprotective agents, they warrant continued study in order to support or disprove this theory. Another similar MAOB inhibitor, rasagiline, is under study in persons with Parkinson's disease. A 2001 report on a study of seventy Parkinson's disease patients found it to be a beneficial drug, similar to selegiline, with improved motor ratings compared to placebo and with a good safety profile. Whether it possesses neuroprotective properties is unknown at the present time.

Dopamine Agonists

The dopamine agonists such as ropinerole and pramipexole that are already FDA-approved are currently being studied in clinical trials with Parkinson's disease patients for possible neuroprotective abilities. In two independent studies (2002) more dopamine brain activity on PET and SPECT scans occurred in persons with Parkinson's disease who took the dopamine agonists ropinerole and pramipexole, compared to those who took carbidopa/levodopa over two and four years, respectively. This suggests that more brain cells survived in persons who took the dopamine agonist medication than those who took carbidopa/levodopa and supports the theory that dopamine agonists may possess neuroprotective properties. Similarly, *in vitro* studies examining dopamine brain cells in a laboratory have shown that dopamine agonists protect the dopamine brain cells from toxic agents and allow them to survive longer.

Riluzole

Additional clinical trials are ongoing with other agents including riluzole, which has been approved for the treatment of ALS (amyotrophic lateral sclerosis, or Lou Gehrig's disease). This drug has antiglutamate activity, meaning that it dampens glutamate, a brain chemical that is thought to be toxic to brain cells if it is overactive.

Anti-Excitotoxic Agents

Other anti-excitotoxic agents such as NMDA, AMPA, and nitric oxide synthase (NOS) inhibitors offer new areas of research as potential neuroprotective therapies. One such drug, remacemide (an NMDA antagonist), is being studied for the possible neuroprotective effects in Huntington's disease and Parkinson's disease.

Bioenergetic Treatments

Bioenergetic drugs such as Coenzyme Q10 (CoQ10) that work in the energy source of the cell, the mitochondria, have been studied in animal models of Parkinson's disease. CoQ10 works with complex I in the mitochondria to produce energy, and it has been shown that complex I is underactive in Parkinson's disease. The results of a large multicenter study of CoQ10 should be available in the near future. Other similar agents that might be considered for future study include creatine, ginkgo biloba, nicotinamide, riboflavin, carnitine, and lipoic acid.

Antioxidants such as vitamin C, vitamin E, glutathione, and iron chelators may offer protection of brain cells due to their ability to scavenge free radicals. Although limited studies on the benefits of vitamins C and E have failed to show a neuroprotective effect in the treatment of Parkinson's disease, in modest amounts they are probably safe to take. NADH (nicotinamide adenine dinucleotide hydrogen) is an antioxidant that helps to produce levodopa and dopamine.

A number of clinical studies of NADH in persons with Parkinson's disease have been conducted. Many of these reported improved motor function in Parkinson's disease patients who took it, but most of these were open-label (non-blinded) studies. A randomized, double-blind, placebo-controlled study of ten Parkinson's disease patients taking intravenous NADH showed no significant difference between the placebo (normal saline or salt water) group and the NADH group. Long-term use and safety of NADH for the treatment of Parkinson's disease has not been studied, and it has not been proven to be an effective and safe treatment for Parkinson's disease.

Many patients ask about the use of intravenous glutathione for Parkinson's disease. In theory, because glutathione levels are reduced in Parkinson's disease, and glutathione may protect cell damage from nitrous oxide, it is thought to play a neuroprotective role. However, at the time this book was written, there have been no published results of the use of glutathione in double-blind placebo-controlled studies; however, future studies of this caliber would be able to prove or disprove it as a therapeutic or neuroprotective agent for Parkinson's disease.

Neurotrophic Factors

Neurotrophic factors are agents that help to repair or rescue damaged brain cells and stimulate the cells so that they can grow back or sprout. GDNF (glial-cell-lined–derived neurotrophic factor) has been studied in the animal models of Parkinson's disease and showed repair and resprouting of damaged dopamine brain cells. Human trials with intraventricular GDNF (the GDNF was delivered directly into the spinal fluid of the brain) were not successful, in part due to intolerable side effects and perhaps because the GDNF was not able to get to the brain cells that needed it. New ways of delivering the GDNF directly to the dopamine brain cells are being studied in rat and monkey animal models of Parkinson's disease. This involves using a genetically engineered virus that can be implanted directly into the brain at the site of brain cell injury. There, the virus is capable of producing GDNF. Scientists are perfecting ways to control the GDNF production by the virus such that it can be stopped or restarted by taking a low dose of an antibiotic such as tetracycline. This will allow more control and thus afford the patient protection should the GDNF prove to cause unwanted side effects or to be harmful rather than helpful.

For instance, if a patient with Parkinson's disease had the viral vector put into his or her brain and then took a small dose of tetracycline, the virus would start producing GDNF to hopefully allow damaged brain cells to be rescued and survive. If the patient, however, developed an unexpected side effect, simply stopping the tetracycline would cause the virus to stop producing the GDNF. A study cited at the American Academy of Neurology (2002) of persons with Parkinson's disease involved the delivery of GDNF locally into the brain. Although this was a small unblinded study, the five patients that received GDNF via a mini-pump and cannula that was placed into the brain cells of the putamen (where the dopamine cells of the SNc project to) improved in their motor function. They experienced marked reductions in "off" time and dyskinesia and increased "on" time after twelve months.

Other similar neurotrophic growth factors are being evaluated in similar studies. These include fibroblast growth factor (FGF), ciliary neurotrophic growth factor (CNGF), brain-derived neurotrophic factor (BDNF) and immunophilins. Immunophilins are proteins that react with certain immuno-suppressant medicines (often used to treat cancer or auto-immune disorders). Some of the immunophilins can stimulate brain cell growth. This has been shown to occur in animal models of Parkinson's disease (rat and monkey MPTP) with a particular immunophilin, GPI-1046. In the MPTP treated monkeys that were treated with GPI-1046, regrowth of MPP+ damaged dopamine neurons occurred, and this regrowth was correlated with improved motor function, such as walking and climbing. Future studies of GPI-1046 and many of these neurotrophic factors in persons with Parkinson's disease will likely occur once these therapies prove to be safe and effective in the animal models.

GM1 Ganglioside

GM1 ganglioside (GM1) is a chemical that forms part of the cell membrane, the part of the cell covering that protects the cell. Scientists have shown GM1 helps injured dopamine cells to recover. A study with the Parkinson's disease monkey model showed the monkeys' motor symptoms significantly decreased and reverted to normal after treatment with GM1 for six to eight weeks. In addition, sprouting or growth of the dopamine nerves along with an increase in dopamine levels was observed. A subsequent double-blind, placebo-controlled study of forty-five people with Parkinson's disease was reported in 1998 by Schneider. GM1 or a placebo was given for sixteen weeks. A significant improvement in muscle rigidity and bradykinesia—slowed movement—was noted in the GM1 group compared to the placebo group. Dr. Schneider and his research team at Thomas Jefferson University in Philadelphia have reported that fifteen of these patients have continued to take GM1 for over four years and that eleven out of the fifteen have better motor function scores than they had four years ago. This research group is now studying the effects of GM1 use over five years in persons with Parkinson's disease. Parkinson's patients and practitioners anxiously await the results.

Minocycline

Minocycline is a semisynthetic tetracycline antibiotic that was reported at the National Academy of Sciences in 2001 to have neuroprotective effects on dopamine brain cells in the rat MPTP model of Parkinson's disease. Minocycline appears to inhibit nitrous oxide (NO) neurotoxicity and MPP+ neurotoxicity. This raises the possibility of neuroprotective tetracyclines for the treatment of Parkinson's disease.

Caffeine

Caffeine intake has been observed to be associated with a lower occurrence of Parkinson's disease. A recent study with the MPTP mouse model of Parkinson's disease showed that mice that were pretreated with caffeine had greater survival of dopamine cells, suggesting that caffeine may have a neuroprotective effect. Caffeine is thought to bind to adenosine receptors in the brain and block their activity. Similar results were obtained with administration of a drug that blocked the A2a adenosine receptor, and genetically engineered mice that lacked this A2a adenosine receptor were resistant to MPTP toxicity. Novel drugs that block these receptors and have similar properties to caffeine may prove to be neuroprotective of dopamine brain cells.

❖ ALTERNATIVE THERAPIES

The line between what is considered "alternative" and conventional is becoming less clear over time. The use of supplements such as NADH, CoQ10, and glutathione, which were discussed at greater length in chapter 8, may, with further study, become the conventional treatments of the future, as more formal research methods prove them effective.

It's important that future research into the prevention and treatment of Parkinson's disease examine a wide range of nontraditional treatments, in order to prove whether they are effective. Therapies that should be examined include antioxidants; herbs; touch therapies such as massage and Reiki; mind-body techniques such as hypnosis, imagery, and meditation; Eastern exercises such as t'ai chi and yoga; Traditional Chinese Medicine and acupuncture; and much more. This is especially true with herbs, which have the potential to interact with medicines and cause unwanted side effects.

There is clearly an interest among persons with Parkinson's disease in using these complementary treatments, as noted in the journal *Neurology*, which reported on findings that 40 percent of 201 patients surveyed used at least one alternative therapy for their Parkinson's disease. The most commonly used were vitamins, herbs, massage, and acupuncture. Clearly, there is a need for placebo-controlled, blind studies of alternative therapies for treatment of Parkinson's disease.

❖ NEUROSURGERY

Surgical therapies will likely involve continued study of deep brain stimulation and lesioning techniques such as pallidotomy, to examine long-term benefits as well as side effects and complications, and to prove what sites of the brain are the best for placing an electrode.

Dr. Rajish Pahwa, director of the Parkinson Center at Kansas University, has some thoughts about the future:

> More patients will be getting surgery in the future, probably 20 percent of all Parkinson's disease patients. Deep brain stimulation (DBS) of the subthalamic nucleus (STN) will be the most preferred procedure, and there will be a shift from doing surgery in advanced disease to moderate disease. There will be improvements in surgical techniques and people might use frameless surgery. Targeting the site for surgical placement of the electrode will improve because of better computer software. IPGs (impulse generators, the battery source for the electrode) will be made by several companies, and they will improve tremendously, just like cardiac pacemakers! The majority of patients don't realize that stem cell use is years and years away, and DBS of the STN at the present time is the best form of treatment to improve the quality of life in patients who

cannot be adequately managed with Parkinson's disease medicines alone.

Tissue transplantation will continue to be researched, although the widespread use of tissue transplants is probably unlikely to occur in the near future as they are still considered to be experimental. Human fetal brain cell transplants have not overall been accepted as a viable, effective therapy, and face ethical concerns from among lawmakers and a divided public.

The recent reports of porcine (pig) fetal tissue transplants showed a small benefit to the patients who received the porcine tissue transplants. However, those who underwent sham (fake) surgery by having a burr hole drilled in the skull, but nothing transplanted into the brain, had similar benefits. Ten persons with Parkinson's disease received porcine dopamine brain transplants and eight received sham surgery, and eighteen months after surgery, both the porcine and sham surgery groups showed a modest, similar improvement in motor function scores. While there are some anecdotal reports from patients and practitioners who claim to have seen marked improvements due to this procedure, it requires extensive further study before it can be recommended as a treatment for Parkinson's patients in general.

Other tissues that might provide a source of dopamine cells include the retina and carotid body. Abstract reports from the Fourteenth International Congress on Parkinson's Disease (2001) suggest that both of these sources have the potential to restore dopamine cell activity in the brain of persons with Parkinson's disease, although the numbers of patients were small (six in each study), there were no control groups, and the results are very preliminary without long-term follow-up assessment.

Neurostem cells for tissue transplantation in humans with Parkinson's disease is a very hot topic in the news. The reality, however, is that stem cell transplants are many years and possibly decades away from being a real therapeutic option for the treatment of Parkinson's disease. Neurostem cells are primitive cells found in embryos; they have not yet developed into more specific cells and thus have the potential to be programmed to become a particular type of cell, such as a dopamine-producing neuron. In theory, these neurostem cells might be a future source of tissue brain transplants for Parkinson's disease or other neurodegenerative conditions. Such cells can be found in the lining of the fluid system (ventricles) of each person's brain, as well as in bone marrow and in human and animal embryos.

The challenge is to teach these primitive cells to become the desired cell, and then for it to survive after being transplanted into the brain and form proper connections, ultimately replacing damaged tissue. Scientists at the University of Wisconsin at Madison and the University of Bonn published results in late 2001 in the journal *Nature Biotechnology* showing that after being transplanted into the brains of baby mice, human stem cells were able to differentiate into specific brain cells (neurons and astrocytes). This is very exciting news, but people with Parkinson's disease need to understand that a huge amount of subsequent research needs to be performed to perfect and understand this technology before it can be tried in human beings. We do not know whether the transplanted cells will survive for long periods of time, or whether they will grow too rapidly into a tumor, or whether they will make the right connections to the damaged cells, or whether other unforseen serious problems might occur after they are transplanted.

❖ GENETICS

Research in the field of genetics will continue to involve many different areas and play a critical role in discovering both the causes of Parkinson's disease and future treatments. Continued study of specific genes that cause familial forms of Parkinson's disease and of the proteins that the genes make will likely provide additional clues as to what leads to dopamine cell death. The example of the mutations found in the alpha-synuclein gene (chromosome number 4) in familial Parkinson's disease, discussed earlier in this chapter, provides an excellent illustration.

Another family with Parkinson's disease was found to have a gene mutation that involves the formation of the protein ubiquitin, which, as previously discussed, helps to break down unwanted or old proteins by tagging them and presenting them to protesomes. This process is mediated by other enzymes called E-ligases. The parkin gene on chromosome number 6 codes for the formation of the protein parkin, which is an E-ligase. A report in the journal *Science* suggests that alpha-synuclein, ubiquitin, and parkin may all interact in the formation of abnormal cell protein clumping, or aggregation, and may be causally linked to dopamine cell death in Parkinson's disease. In another, similar report, dopamine cell loss with inclusion bodies in the SNc occurred in rats when scientists caused disruption of the ubiquitin-protesomal system.

These three inherited forms of Parkinson's disease, although they represent a relatively small number of families where a single gene is responsible for the cause of Parkinson's disease, may greatly improve our understanding of what causes Parkinson's disease at the cellular level. In other words, we are beginning to more fully understand what actually occurs within the dopamine cell itself that results in cell injury and subsequent death.

Another contribution from these familial genetic forms of Parkinson's disease is the ability to develop genetic animal models of Parkinson's disease. One example of this is the newly genetically engineered alpha-synuclein *Drosophilia* fruit fly. By overexpressing alpha-synuclein, researchers were able to create flies with Parkinson's disease. These flies show clinical evidence of Parkinson's disease (i.e, they have difficulty performing normal fly motor behavior such as hanging upside down from the lid of a jar). This motor function improves after the flies drink sugar solution with levodopa. And upon postmortem examination of these flies, loss of dopamine brain cells and inclusions that appear similar to Lewy bodies have been found.

According to Dr. Matt Farrer, director of Neurogenetics at the Mayo Clinic in Jacksonville, Florida:

> This new animal model of Parkinson's disease and others like it provide powerful tools that will reveal additional clues about what causes Parkinson's disease and help define new effective therapies for humans.

Other susceptibility genes that predispose persons to the development of Parkinson's disease will most likely be found. These gene variants exist in many persons and may need a trigger in the form of a toxin or a stress to the body—such as infection, inflammation, or suppression of the immune system—for the gene and its protein product to be expressed and for Parkinson's disease to develop.

It appears that the genetic causes of Parkinson's disease are polygenic, meaning that many different genes exist as the cause of familial Parkinson's disease. Ultimately, the so-called "sporadic" form of Parkinson's disease may in fact turn out to be genetically caused after all. A recent study reported in the *Journal of the American Medical Association* of 174 families with a diagnosis of idiopathic or sporadic Parkinson's disease in one identified patient who had at least one reported family member with Parkinson's disease supports this concept. This study suggested five different genetic factors (chromosomes 5, 6, 8, 9, and 17) were linked to Parkinson's disease. A total of 870 family members were studied, with 378 having been diagnosed with Parkinson's disease, 379 who were without symptoms or signs of Parkinson's disease, and 113 who were without a certain diagnosis. The parkin gene on chromosome 6 was found in many families where at least one person had the onset of Parkinson's disease before age 40, and families with typical late-onset Parkinson's disease were found to have genetic markers on chromosomes 5, 8, 9, and 17.

Another pivotal study, performed by the company DE-CODE in Iceland, found evidence to support that chromosome number 1 is the cause of Parkinson's disease. This study is very unique in that it was able to look at 772 persons—both living and deceased—who were diagnosed with Parkinson's disease over the prior fifty years and over eleven generations, using computerized genealogic information on 610,920 Icelandic people. The goal of the study was to determine whether these 772 persons were more likely to be related to one another, suggesting a genetic role for Parkinson's disease. The study did find that persons with the disease diagnosed at age 50 or later were much more likely to be related to one another than controls (age matched without a diagnosis), with a risk of Parkinson's disease equaling 6.7 times greater for siblings, 3.2 times greater for children, and 2.7 times greater for nieces or nephews. This study supports a genetic component for late-onset Parkinson's disease that was previously diagnosed as sporadic—not inherited—Parkinson's disease. This gives credence to the idea that familial or genetically determined Parkinson's disease is probably grossly underestimated due to underreporting and underdiagnosis. Similar studies in other countries will be needed to see if this theory holds up. PROGENI (Parkinson's Research: The Organized Genetics Initiative) is a study that is under way and will eventually collect over four hundred pairs of siblings (sisters and brothers) with Parkinson's disease in order to study genetic risk factors.

Another area where genetics is playing a role in the world of Parkinson's disease research is in the development of genetically engineered viruses. These viruses are modified by inserting genes so that they can produce certain factors such as neurotrophic agents (e.g., GDNF) that stimulate regrowth of dopamine nerves, or enzymes (e.g., tyrosine hydroxylase) that promote dopamine production. These genetically modified viruses can be delivered directly to the injured brain cells through surgical techniques, in order to stimulate growth and survival of dopamine cells and increase dopamine activity. Neurostem cells have very recently been used in a similar way. Rather than using them as a direct tissue brain transplant, scientists have been able to use genes to make the stem cells produce the neurotrophic factor GDNF and have shown it to protect dopamine brain cells from dying in the 6-hydroxydopamine mouse model of Parkinson's disease.

Overall, then, genetics will play an important future role in Parkinson's disease, through

- Identification of single genes for familial Parkinson's disease;

- Identification of susceptibility genes that increase a person's risk for Parkinson's disease;
- Identification of proteins made by these genes and the function of these proteins in order to learn more about what causes dopamine cell death;
- Development of genetic animal models of Parkinson's disease;
- Development of genetically modified viruses and neurostem cells to deliver trophic and neuroprotective factors directly to dopamine cells; and
- Development of drugs that alter gene expression to slow the progression of the disease in genetic Parkinson's disease models.

Dr. Matt Farrer's hope is that all the genes will be identified and that this data will be integrated together into a comprehensive molecular understanding of this disease. Says Dr. Farrer:

> The future direction in genetics is the way of the twenty-first century—genetic research is opening novel avenues of investigation never before imagined. It will lead to palliative remedies and prevention in individuals determined to be at risk for the development of Parkinson's disease.

❖ EPIDEMIOLOGY AND ENVIRONMENTAL FACTORS

Epidemiological studies can provide clues as to which factors predispose one to getting Parkinson's disease and which factors may protect someone from getting the disease. Most of the risk factors outlined in chapter 2 were identified by such studies. Because Parkinson's disease is most likely caused by multiple factors and probably requires the interaction of genetic and environmental factors, it is extremely important that risk factors for Parkinson's disease continue to be sought. The recent reports on the relationship of caffeine, nicotine, and estrogens to Parkinson's disease may eventually have a profound impact on the understanding of what causes or protects against dopamine cell death and lead to effective new treatments. Prospective studies over many years that examine people who have not yet been diagnosed with Parkinson's disease are sorely needed, as well as case-control studies that compare persons with Parkinson's disease to people who do not have the condition, to better identify and isolate these risk factors.

◆ FUTURE ECONOMICS AND HEALTH CARE NEEDS

As the population in America continues to age, the number of people with Parkinson's disease will grow considerably. Over one million Americans currently have Parkinson's disease, and these numbers will increase substantially as the American population ages.

Hence, this increased number of Parkinson's patients will bring with them a need for improved medical care, including financial assistance in covering the cost of prescription medicines. They will also need caregivers and assistance for home care, as well as rehabilitative therapists to provide physical, occupational, and speech therapy. Assisted-living and nursing-home care will be required by this growing population of patients, as will surgical centers specializing in Parkinson's. Finally, more doctors and nurses who specialize in Parkinson's will be needed as well.

In addition to the increased economic and health care needs of an ever-growing Parkinson's disease population, the greater demand for research dollars will also need to be met. Hopefully, this will occur. In April of 2000, the National Institutes of Health's Dr. Gerald Fischbach presented its Parkinson's disease research agenda to Congress. The NIH report recommended an increase of $71.4 million for the first year and $947 million over five years. Such leadership by top researchers and national organizations, as well as celebrities like Michael J. Fox, is essential in the fight for financial support for continued research. The future truly depends upon the success of productive research to find better treatments, to identify risks and potential causes of Parkinson's disease, to find neuroprotective agents that may prevent Parkinson's disease, and ultimately, to seek a cure.

❖ HOW CAN YOU HELP?

First, Parkinson's patients can consider joining one of the patient organizations whose mission is to aid patients by disseminating and exchanging information and supporting further research. Membership will provide many benefits, in the form of newsletters, support groups, and other information and interaction that will help you optimize your own health, but at the same time, it provides critical mass for national efforts.

Second, you can provide financial support to organizations that are actively working to promote research into Parkinson's disease. Appendix A of this book lists a variety of worthy organizations that will make your donation work on behalf of Parkinson's patients everywhere.

You can also consider participating in studies or clinical trials. Without the participation of people with Parkinson's disease, researchers cannot test the safety and effectiveness of therapies. Because there are so many people with Parkinson's disease, it might sound easy to find enough patients to participate in clinical studies, but this is not always the case. If you do have Parkinson's disease and you are interested in being involved in clinical studies, discuss it with your physician and contact some of the national organizations listed in Appendix A, as well as the National Institutes of Health, for more information.

Before you participate in a study or trial, however, there are some important questions to ask:

- What is the purpose of the study? What is it trying to prove?
- Is it approved by an IRB (internal review board)? This ensures that it is a safe and regulated study that strives to protect the patient from any possible harm.
- How long is the study and what specifically does it require of you? For example, do you need to have blood drawn? How many visits to the study site do you need to make? Do you need to be examined or perform special motor or mental tasks?
- Is it a blinded or placebo-controlled study? (You may be put on a placebo or the study drug and not know which you are taking.)
- What adverse events might occur? (Could you have a side effect from the study drug?)
- Is there any monetary or other reward for participation? (Some studies provide reimbursement for travel or provide free samples of the study drug after it is completed if it is FDA-approved.)

- Whom do I contact if I have questions or a problem while I am in the study?
- Can I withdraw from the study? (The answer to this question should always be yes; you have the right as a patient to withdraw from any study at any time and for whatever reason.)

Another key point is that you should never participate in any study without giving written consent saying that you understand the purpose and details of the study and volunteer to participate. More details about clinical studies can be found on the NIH Web site: http://clinicaltrials.gov.

❖ THE FUTURE

The future of Parkinson's disease is brighter than ever. There is no doubt that continued research by an ever-growing international team of scientists will continue to put together additional pieces of the puzzle, and one by one, as the pieces fit together, the picture will become clearer. It will be a picture of better drugs, better surgery, holistic approaches, possible causes, neuroprotection, and slowing of the disease—a picture of health and wellness, a picture of a better world.

The Power of the Mind and Spirit on Illness

In the stillness of my soul, it is there I know I am a spiritual being, one with God and everything.

—*Jill Marjama-Lyons*

According to religious science minister Brian Langlois, the word *disease* comes from *dis* meaning "without" or "not," and *ease,* meaning "harmony" or "balance." So *dis-ease* means without harmony, out of balance, or ill at ease. When we are ill at ease or out of balance—be it due to a loss of dopamine neurons, cancer, a cold, or emotional or spiritual stress—we need to correct the problem that is causing the dis-ease and restore balance to our mind, body, and spirit.

There are so many ways we can achieve this: through traditional therapies such as medications and surgery, and through alternative therapies such as acupuncture, herbs, vitamins, and t'ai chi.

But in this closing chapter, I want to touch upon one way that is within everyone's own control: the role of spirit and attitude, and how our spirituality—however you define it—can play a role in our wellness.

We are all spiritual beings, and as such we all have a connection to one another, to God—whether you view God religiously or more in the sense of a universal energy or life force—and all living things. Many of us, myself included, are not as fully in touch with our spiritual selves as we could be. We get easily caught up in our busy, frantic world—the world that says buy groceries, pay bills, clean the kitchen, feed the cat, walk the dog, make dinner, go to work, go to the doctor, take your medicine, exercise, and so on.

We may pause to pray or go to some type of religious service as part of our schedule and as an attempt to connect to our spiritual selves. But ultimately, how many of us truly feel, cultivate, and experience our spiritual nature completely on an ongoing daily basis?

This tendency can be dangerous when dealing with a physical condition or illness such as Parkinson's disease. If we—whether patient, caregiver, doctor, nurse, family member, or friend—concentrate only on the physical illness and physical symptoms and forget to acknowledge the emotional, psychological, and spiritual self, we are not allowing ourselves to treat the person with Parkinson's disease wholly. More importantly, we are ignoring and preventing perhaps the most important channel for healing and obtaining optimal health.

Spirituality can mean many different things. When discussing spirituality, this book refers to the nonphysical part of ourselves, the part deep inside that we cannot see or touch, that makes us alive and life worth living. This includes all our thoughts, hopes, dreams, and desires, as well as our emotions and our relationships to people, animals, nature, and a higher power such as God or the universe.

Sonya says it well.

I have continued to grow in awareness of my spiritual nature. In fact, getting Parkinson's disease has helped me to do so. I realize that the body I inhabit is only a small part of me, and if I tremor or am a little slower, it doesn't change who I am on the inside. I used to be one of those type A personalities, and Parkinson's disease has taught me to slow down and enjoy the simple pleasures. I spend more time sitting on my front porch looking at my beautiful flowers and listening to the birds. My husband Jack and I hold hands and hug more and smile at each other more. It might sound corny, but I am seeing the world through new eyes and I am closer to my husband and God thanks to Parkinson's disease.

The power of faith, prayer, love, and hope is immeasurable. In fact, Western medicine is just now starting to catch up with this idea, something that Eastern medicine has known for thousands of years. Medical studies have shown that women who had metastatic breast cancer who participated in regular group therapy lived longer than the women who did not participate. The communion with the other women gave them hope, comfort, emotional support, and companionship, which had a positive impact on their physical health. Other studies have shown a reduced risk of recurrent heart disease in patients with known heart disease who adopted a new lifestyle that included meditation, yoga, exercise, and a healthier diet. Qi gong, a healing form of t'ai chi practiced by many Chinese as a part of their daily lives, has been shown to increase life expectancy in Chinese patients with cancer. Duke University researchers have reported that patients with rheumatoid arthritis have been able to cope better with pain as a result of their daily spiritual experiences. And in one surprising blinded study, infertility patients who were prayed for were shown to have substantially higher rates of successful pregnancy than patients who were not the focus of the prayers.

Learning to tap into our spiritual selves and world is a highly personal endeavor, which will differ among all individuals. Ways to begin this process include exploring one's faith and belief in a higher power or God. Some ways to accomplish this can include

- Attending religious services;
- Reading books about faith, prayer, spirituality, and religion;
- Talking to others about their faith;
- Spending more time with nature, such as sitting in a garden, walking by a river or beach, or listening to the rain;
- Petting a dog or cat;
- Hugging a friend or loved one;
- Holding someone's hands and looking into his or her eyes; and
- Listening to inspirational music.

The many mind-body therapies, such as meditation, prayer, yoga, and other approaches discussed in chapter 7, are also ways to help connect to a spiritual self and/or achieve the relaxation response.

Ultimately, the list of ways to connect with our spiritual selves is endless. But the important thing is to acknowledge that this part of our being indeed exists and needs attention every day, just as much as our physical selves do. Daily treatment of your spirit is just as important as your daily medication or daily exercise.

❖ HEALING THROUGH POSITIVE THOUGHT

The power of faith, prayer, and positive thoughts can be miraculous in some cases. We have all heard of people who had cancer and simply refused to accept it, and, who then, to the amazement of the doctors, recovered completely. I have had a similar experience with one of my patients.

After Joe moved to Florida, he came to see me for the first time. He had been diagnosed with Parkinson's disease almost twenty years before. His wife, Faye, said right away to me, "Doctor, my husband is a miracle—I have been praying his Parkinson's away and I think he will be the first person to be cured through prayer." She really believed this, and he smiled lovingly at her, as though she were right in a sort of matter-of-fact way. I smiled and thought they were sweet, and that their faith and love had probably had a positive effect on his illness, but I didn't really believe he would be cured. I couldn't dismiss the possibility either, however, because of Joe and Faye's bold, unrelenting belief that this was what would happen. Faye even went so far as to say that she wanted me to consider doing a special dopamine PET scan in the future, when his Parkinson's disease symptoms will have stopped completely, to show that it is normal. Joe is currently on low doses of medication and his physical exam is consistent with mild Parkinson's disease, which is very rare for someone who has had symptoms for over twenty years. Both Joe and Faye swear that he has improved in his physical condition over the past five years.

Is this faith, or is it the power of the mind to heal the body? Is it the benefits of nutrition combined with the right medications? Or is it a combination of all these factors? I have many other patients who have had Parkinson's disease for fifteen to thirty years, and although they have more advanced disease than Joe, they are all living independent, high-quality lives. One may argue these patients just have a milder form of Parkinson's disease, that they're simply lucky.

But I do not believe this is so. What I believe and have found, in working with over a thousand patients with Parkinson's disease, is that the patients who are coping the best—even with advanced Parkinson's disease—are positive in their thinking, have a strong faith in a higher spiritual being, and have healthy, loving relationships. They are connected with their spiritual selves and are allowing their spirituality to positively influence their physical health and daily lives.

Bob, a 57-year-old accountant, now retiring due to disability from Parkinson's disease, feels that his faith is a continual source of strength.

> I pray daily, many times, and I am learning to focus on the important things in my life. Early retirement has allowed me more time to spend with my children and wife and to volunteer at our church and at the Parkinson center. I find this very rewarding. I try to stay focused on the good that has come out of this and to accept that I have some limitations with my physical functions, but that each day is a gift that I intend to use well.

Sam, a 45-year-old teacher, says that in one respect, Parkinson's disease hasn't changed his life at all.

> I still have the choice of choosing my attitude. . . . It is my attitude that determines whether the changes resulting from Parkinson's disease are negative or positive changes. My belief in God and my associated faith in

him have been and continue to be the most significant determining factor in the quality of my entire life, including the past three years with Parkinson's disease. I believe God has a plan for me, which happens to include this bout with Parkinson's disease. My goal is to conform my plan for my life to his plan. I also believe I have a purpose for being here. My quest is to discover that purpose and to fulfill it. Parkinson's disease does not change the plan or purpose of my life, it only provides an added dimension to the journey.

Spirituality exists in everyone and is everywhere, and it is perhaps most profound when experienced between two or more living beings. I try to be very positive with my patients. I pray for guidance from God in the actions I take and the words I choose with my patients, so that I can help them however I am supposed to. I am not perfect; I have my bad days like anyone else, and sometimes I wonder if I am really helping anyone or really making a difference. Like many doctors, I tend to focus primarily on what I can do for my patients, but I realize every so often that my patients are probably doing more for me, and teaching me more than I know.

John is a 72-year-old retired architect who at his last visit with me looked me in the eye and said, "Doctor, you aren't going to leave, are you? I feel so good when I see you, I get all emotional." Tears welled up in his eyes. I was silent for a moment, then tears welled up in my eyes. Did he have any idea how wonderful he made me feel? I tried to tell him by replying, "I'm not going anywhere. Whenever I get discouraged or tired or think I should change my career, God sends someone like you to say something like that, and then I know I'm right where I'm supposed to be."

This was a spiritual experience; there was a deep connection between John and me, an understanding of needing and caring for one another.

◈ THE POWER OF YOUR THOUGHTS

Some faiths believe that all thoughts are prayers and that our thoughts directly affect body function, right down to the basic human cell that makes up all of our organs. Some faiths believe that cells have memory and can be programmed by our thoughts and beliefs, so that healthy positive thoughts will promote healthy cells, organs, and body function, and negative unhealthy thoughts will do the reverse. This idea may seem too far-fetched for many to embrace; however, we all can relate to our thoughts programming or dictating our behavior.

For instance, if you fully believe that you will miss the bus, and then you procrastinate and wander around the house looking for your keys and bag and then are late in getting to the bus stop, was it your belief that led you to miss the bus and influenced your behavior, or are you just a victim of bad circumstance? This is the self-fulfilling prophecy. What you believe can become your reality and dictate your behavior, to then make your belief come true. Robert Bitzer makes this point in his book *Collected Essays of Robert Bitzer*, in the chapter "Belief Comes First."

> Demonstration is very simple, but it involves very definite mental laws. It responds to your belief. It heals according to your belief. It prospers you according to your belief. Your belief becomes the very thing you think about. As long as you believe that you cannot, your belief holds you back. As you change your belief, the conditions around you change.

Have you been paying attention to your thoughts lately? What are you thinking regarding your health? Are you angry, fearful of becoming disabled and a burden to your family, or worse yet, do you think you have been given a death sentence because you were diagnosed with Parkinson's disease? These may be natural initial emotions and thoughts when you are first diagnosed with any physical illness. However, if these thoughts persist, you run the danger of negatively influencing your behavior and health. If you do not have hope, you may not seek out health care professionals who truly understand Parkinson's disease, and thus you may not optimize your treatment. You may not exercise, and you may withdraw from social activities and become seriously depressed.

This is one of the challenges I face as a physician: to convince patients and their caregivers to be positive in the face of a physical illness, to continue to pursue life on all levels, and to not give in to the disease and let it control them.

Rita and Bob were an elderly couple, married for fifty years after being childhood sweethearts. Rita was diagnosed with Parkinson's disease in her early sixties, and after eight years, she began struggling with her motor function. She had bad tremors that did not respond to the medication, and her movements were either too slow or too fast due to dyskinesia. Bob had to help her with almost everything, including dressing, bathing, and getting up out of a chair, and sometimes he had to feed her. She could walk slowly with a cane, and during her two hours of good, "on" time, she was independent. She was alert and had no difficulty with her thinking. But she was depressed. Bob was depressed but wouldn't admit it, and carried on as a dedicated husband. Rita and Bob struggled greatly because of how Parkinson's disease had affected their lives. They stopped going to the theater, an activity they had always loved.

They stopped socializing with their friends, except for religious services, and spent most of their time simply caring for Rita. The focus of their lives became Rita's Parkinson's disease.

Some of this you might say was unavoidable, but much of it was not. They could have gone for counseling, which I recommended many times, to learn how to better cope. This might have given Bob permission to pursue his golf interest and to leave Rita with a friend or family member for four hours once or twice a week. They might have realized that they could still go to the theater: Rita might have tremors or dyskinesia, but they could get seats in the back row or balcony area, where her wheelchair would allow her to be more comfortable and manage among the crowd. You may recognize Rita and Bob from chapter 6. They have struggled, but have made tremendous gains since.

Andy's story starts out the same as Rita's but has a very different ending. Andy first came to see me at age 58. He was diagnosed with Parkinson's disease at age 50. Like Rita, Andy was married and had had Parkinson's disease for eight years. He suffered from a debilitating slow time during which it was difficult to do simple motor tasks like walking and writing. Like Rita, he frequently had violent uncontrollable dyskinesia of his arms and legs and had few good "on" times. However, unlike Rita, he continued to work full-time as a meteorologist, he continued to fly-fish regularly, he kept up with his friends socially, and he was not depressed. He could have easily have gotten early retirement due to medical disability. Instead, he asked his boss to give him the late evening shift, when less people were around and the demands were less, so that he could effectively accomplish his work. He would take his medication as frequently as every hour and at lower doses in order to function better while at work. He loved fly-fishing and refused to stop, despite having disabling motor symptoms from Parkinson's disease. I remember smiling with him as he talked about fly-fishing and how he had gotten stuck once in the middle of the stream while having an "off" period due to the Parkinson's and had to wait thirty minutes for his medication to kick in before he could move again and then retrieve the fish he had landed. He reassured me that he fly-fishes in shallow water!

It amazes me that two people with almost the exact same stage of Parkinson's disease and degree of motor difficulty can lead such different lives. Why is this? The answer is simple: It is the different belief system and attitude of the patient that dictates and determines his or her behavior. Andy's refusal to let Parkinson's disease change his life adversely led him to continue to fish and work and pursue life as best he could. These things fed his soul, gave him pleasure, and tended to his spiritual self.

J. Kennedy Shultz addresses the power of our thoughts in his book *You Are the Power: A Guide to Personal Greatness*:

> We must understand that the power of mind is both the power that binds us and the power that can just as easily set us free. . . . We can take absolute charge of our own thinking and create a consciousness dominated by healthy ideas. We can do this in spite of what the world around us says we ought to believe or ought to expect. No one can put us in charge of our thoughts except ourselves. And no one can block our access to our own creative thinking.

Becky was a former nurse who retired early because of Parkinson's disease. Because she was a nurse, you would think that she would have been very proactive in her care, but in fact she did not keep her doctor's appointments. She would run out of her medication for her Parkinson's symptoms, and only because the doctor would not refill them because she hadn't been to the clinic for almost a year, would she make an appointment. This was her routine for four years, but then something changed. She started going to a Parkinson's support group and started to attend the group's yoga and t'ai chi classes. She started taking her medication. Within months I saw the transformation of Becky into the happier, more vibrant person she once was, the one I had heard about from other nurses in the hospital. I asked her what was different.

> I thought I knew more about Parkinson's disease because I was a nurse, but what I knew was from nursing school in the 1960s, that Parkinson's disease was a horrible illness and that I would end up in a nursing home and not be able to take care of myself, so why should I care or try? I was very wrong. Attending the support group let me learn that there are many good treatments, and I saw that people who had Parkinson's disease for over fifteen years were still walking and living good lives. I found hope and after I started taking my medications and keeping my appointments, I felt better, I could move better. I have even gotten involved in a study with a new drug for Parkinson's.

Becky found hope. Her thoughts about Parkinson's disease, which were not only negative but wrong, had severely hampered her treatment for the first four years. Her renewed hope and change in her thinking led her to change her behavior and improve her self-care and self-worth.

J. Kennedy Schultz further emphasizes the importance of having healthy thoughts in the following passage:

We do not heal disease. We get rid of it by getting beyond it. Healing is about establishing health, not about destroying disease or anything else. All mental healing begins with the establishment of a healthy idea in the consciousness of the individual, a healthy idea about the part of one's physical being that is now suffering from illness, a healthy idea about life in general, a healthy idea about one's life in particular, and one's body in general.

❖ THE VOICES OF PATIENTS

Here are some quotes from patients who, while challenged by the condition, have continued to live well, thanks to their attitude, a focus on the positive, and a connection to their spirit.

Parkinson's disease has strengthened my faith in God and taught me how precious life is and to live every day to its fullest. Sure, I have tremors and I am a little slower, but since being diagnosed with Parkinson's disease, I have cut my work hours and am spending more time with my wife and children and enjoying life more than ever.

—John

Parkinson's disease has made a big change in my life. I appreciate and value things more now. Retirement came earlier; we bought a motor home and have made long-delayed travel plans. We adjusted very well.

—David

The bright side of having Parkinson's disease is all the nice people I have met. The support group is great. Belief in God plays a big factor in just getting through the day and knowing he is always there for me.

—Al

Many good things have come out of having Parkinson's disease. Quitting work has allowed me time to do some things I want to do, such as volunteering, which I did not previously have the time to do. Another good thing is my wife went to work to help provide for the family. The timing was right for this move, as she had spent the past twenty-four years as a full-time mom raising the kids and was unsure of herself in getting a job. The disability I had from Parkinson's disease created a necessity that gave her the boost she needed to make the transition. In addition to this, other by-products of this disease are that I have slowed my pace down and begun to enjoy and appreciate all the good things in life . . . parts of my life that have always been there, but was previously too busy to notice.

—Dan

I was in denial for a good five years. I just didn't want to believe it. I was 58 years old and living my life just fine when whammo, you got Parkinson's disease, that's why you shake and trip on the shag carpet. It's taken me a good ten years to come to grips with the whole deal. I can now see that at age 68 I'm really not that bad off compared to a lot of other 68-year-olds. In fact I'm actually a lot healthier than my buddies. One died from a heart attack, another had prostate cancer, and another has pretty bad arthritis. They're actually jealous of me because all I have is Parkinson's disease and

I shake a little and I'm really not much slower than they are. Some diseases don't have any effective treatments; there are really good medicines that help me move better, so I am lucky. When I started counting my blessings and stopped moping about having Parkinson's disease, I got back to my old happy-go-lucky self, it took a good eight years, but I did it. I think talking to my friends and learning more about Parkinson's disease and the good treatments for it helped me a lot. It's not the end of the world like I first thought it was. Life is good and I appreciate that I am still here and I have a lot more living to do.

—Howard

◆ MOVING FORWARD

And so, as we come to the conclusion, it is my belief, my prayer, my hope, my dream, and my desire that all of us will learn to explore our spiritual nature and cultivate this part of ourselves in order to unleash its power to help us live more harmonious, balanced, and healthy lives.

> When we are healed
> We are not healed alone
> We bless our brothers and sisters
> That they may be healed with us
> As we are healed with them
> —*A Course in Miracles*

Appendix A
Parkinson's Disease Resources

ABOUT THE INTERNET

Throughout this resources section, there are references to various Web sites and Internet-based resources. The Internet is a valuable resource where patients, family members, and health care professionals can exchange ideas and information about Parkinson's disease. If you have access to the Internet, you can access this book's own Web site at http://www.docjill.com, as well as the many sites referenced in this section. If you are not familiar with the Internet, visit your local library and ask the librarian to teach you how to access sites on its computers. A word of caution: When reading anything on the Internet, know the source of information and do not believe everything you read. Also, whatever you read—whether it's information about a product or a breakthrough treatment or even a cure for Parkinson's disease—be sure to note the source of information (e.g., a newspaper article, medical journal, etc.) so that you can discuss it with your treating physicians and health care providers.

KEY PARKINSON'S ORGANIZATIONS

National Parkinson Foundation, Inc.
Bob Hope Parkinson Research Center
1501 N.W. Ninth Avenue (Bob Hope Road)
Miami, FL 33136-1494
(800) 327-4545 or (305) 547-6666
http://www.parkinson.org
mailbox@parkinson.org

The National Parkinson Foundation began in 1957 as a small therapeutic facility and now spearheads a network of world-class institutions offering expert diagnosis, physical, occupational, speech, and neuropsychological therapies as well as a state-of-the-art research laboratory. In addition, the foundation provides educational and medical information, including the quarterly journal *The Parkinson Report*, for Parkinson's patients, their families, neurologists, and general medical practitioners. Its goal is to find the cause and cure of Parkinson's disease and other neurological disorders, through dedicated research, in our lifetime. The NPF Web site is an excellent resource for general information, free publications, research agendas, and up-to-the-minute news reports. Donations can be made securely online, by phone, or by mail.

The American Parkinson's Disease Association
1250 Hylan Boulevard, Suite 4B
Staten Island, NY 10305-1946
(800) 223-2732 or (718) 981-8001
http://www.apdaparkinson.com
info@apdaparkinson.org

Since 1961, the American Parkinson's Disease Association has been seeking to "Ease the Burden and Find the Cure" for this disease, through education, patient/family support, research, and fund-raising. Monies raised through contributions, direct-mail response, and special events sponsored by the national office and chapters, along with their bequest program and gifts from foundations and corporations, are used for funding their programs. Their ever-expanding resources include written manuals (which have been translated into several languages), a research and treatment newsletter (which is distributed quarterly to over 200,000 addresses), and an annually updated Parkinson's Disease Resource Guide, which is distributed worldwide. All of these resources are free, plus select written material is available to download at their Web site or available on audiotape for a small fee. Not only does the APDA sponsor sixty-five chapters and more than eight hundred support groups, it also funds fifty-three Information and Referral Centers across the country. In addition, the APDA offers information and support to meet the unique needs of the "younger" Parkinson's patient.

Parkinson's Disease Foundation
William Black Medical Building
Columbia-Presbyterian Medical Center

710 West 168th Street
New York, NY 10032-9982
(800) 457-6676 or (212) 923-4700
http://www.pdf.org/index.cfm
info@pdf.org

The Parkinson's Disease Foundation was established in 1957. After a merger with the United Parkinson Foundation, its goal remains to support and promote the highest-quality worldwide research into the cause(s) and cure of Parkinson's disease, and to find better symptomatic treatments, through a variety of internationally supported grant programs. The foundation, which also acts as a liaison between physicians, scientists, and laypersons, sponsors educational symposia and distributes the quarterly-published *PDF News* and the *PDF Science Bulletin*, along with publishing a vast collection of booklets, pamphlets, and individual essays. In addition, persons with Parkinson's disease who call the foundation can speak directly with a staff member to address their needs and concerns, and to receive referrals to supports groups, clinical neurologists, and a variety of nonprofit and for-profit agencies related to their unique needs. Free online registration is available to those seeking to become an active member of the PDF's service communities. Members will receive via e-mail select portions of the quarterly newsletter and the new *Science Bulletin*, along with other carefully selected publications of interest.

Michael J. Fox Foundation for Parkinson's Research
Grand Central Station
P. O. Box 4777
New York, NY 10163
(800) 708-7644
http://www.michaeljfox.org

This organization, founded by actor Michael J. Fox, was created to raise the monies necessary to help researchers meet their attainable goal of finding a cure for Parkinson's disease. Its unique approach to fund-raising includes celebrity auctions and media-based events. Those wishing to donate to MJF can do so by mail or by calling its toll-free number.

World Parkinson Disease Association
Via Zuretti, 35

20125 Milano
Italy
Phone: (39) 02 66713111
http://www.wpda.org/
info@wpda.org

The World Parkinson Disease Association was officially established in 1998, as a result of the joint efforts of the American Parkinson's Disease Association and the Italian Parkinson's Association, who saw the need for the Parkinson world-community to have access to the educational resources available. The two main goals of WPDA are to improve the quality of life of the world Parkinson community through education, and to establish greater cooperation and exchange of communications among the various national patients' organizations. The WPDA's Web site offers the latest information on Parkinson's disease research and provides access to a large variety of articles and publications, which are available in several different languages. Links are provided to the Web sites of their worldwide members.

National Institute of Neurological Disorders and Stroke
NIH Neurological Institute
P.O. Box 5801
Bethesda, MD 20824
(800) 352-9424
http://www.ninds.nih.gov/

The U.S. Congress created the National Institute of Neurological Disorders and Stroke in 1950, as one of the more than two dozen research institutes and centers that comprise the National Institutes of Health (NIH). As stated in their Web site, "The mission of the NINDS is to reduce the burden of neurological disease—a burden borne by every age group, every segment of society, and people all over the world. To accomplish this goal the NINDS supports and conducts research, both basic and clinical, on the normal and diseased nervous system, fosters the training of investigators in the basic and clinical neurosciences, and seeks better understanding, diagnosis, treatment, and prevention of neurological disorders." At the NINDS Web site, you will find information on their funding strategies, along with the latest related news and events. Click "Parkinson's disease" under the list of disorders to find more information on their broad range of studies related directly to this disease.

The Parkinson's Institute

1170 Morse Avenue
Sunnyvale, CA 94089-1605
(408) 734-2800 or (800) 786-2958
http://www.parkinsonsinstitute.org/

The Parkinson's Institute, established in 1982 and incorporated in 1988, is currently one of the largest movement-disorders facilities in the United States. The mission of this not-for-profit organization is "to seek the cause(s) and find a cure for Parkinson's disease; to provide the best available medical care to patients with Parkinson's disease and related movement disorders; to investigate new and more effective diagnostic and treatment methods; and to develop prevention strategies." Patient care, clinical research, and basic research are all conducted at their Sunnyvale, California, center. Monetary donations can be made online through a secure server. Visit their Web site for information regarding the variety of gifting opportunities available and to learn about their Tissue Donation Program (which seeks brain, blood, and cerebrospinal fluid samples needed for research purposes).

Parkinson's Resource Organization

74-090 El Paseo, Suite 102
Palm Desert, CA 92260-4135
(760) 773-5628 or toll-free (877) 775-4111
http://www.parkinsonsresource.org/
copsca@gte.net

Parkinson's Resource Organization, formerly known as Children of Parkinsonians, was established in 1990 by Jo Rosen, a woman whose mother and husband were stricken with Parkinson's disease in the 1980s. The goal of PRO is to educate and emotionally support the families of people with Parkinson's disease, along with raising monies to support respite care for caregivers through an annual celebrity-attended fund-raising event. Support for Parkinson's Resource Organization can be made through a suggested donation for their monthly newsletter, or by contacting PRO directly.

Parkinson's Action Network

300 North Lee Street, Suite 500

Alexandria, VA 22314
(703) 518-8877 or (800) 850-4726
http://www.parkinsonaction.org/
info@parkinsonsaction.org

Parkinson's Action Network was founded by former lawyer Joan I. Samuelson in 1991, four years after she was diagnosed with Parkinson's disease. While focusing on action and advocacy to end Parkinson's disease, the primary and secondary goals of PAN are to promote a level of research support sufficient to produce effective treatments and a cure, and to provide an informed, organized, and effective voice in public-policy issues affecting the search for a cure. PAN strongly encourages Parkinson's disease patients and their other supporters to get involved by writing advocacy letters to their state senators and representatives. Monetary donations, which can be made securely online, will help enable them to continue training and mobilizing advocates, and to further their grassroots lobbying efforts in Washington, D.C.

The Parkinson Alliance
211 College Road East, 3rd floor
Princeton, NJ 08520
(609) 688-0870 or (800) 579-8440
http://www.parkinsonalliance.net/home.html
admin@parkinsonalliance.net

The Parkinson Alliance, established by Margaret Tuchman, a Parkinson's disease patient, and her husband, Martin, was formed to raise money for Parkinson's disease research through private contributions and fund-raising events. According to their Web site, "The Tuchman Foundation currently matches every dollar raised, and the Parkinson Alliance leverage contributions by challenging the major national Parkinson's organizations to match the donations and award pilot study program grants to qualified research projects that will use the money for the initial studies needed to qualify for NIH funding." Donations can be made online, by telephone, or by mail. A subscription to their biannual newsletter is available free of charge.

LISTSERVS AND ONLINE SUPPORT

There are several major listservs—online e-mail–based support groups—for people with Parkinson's disease and their caregivers.

Parkinson's Disease Information Exchange Network/Parkinsn-L List
This unmoderated international forum provides an opportunity for those interested in Parkinson's disease—including patients and caregivers—to exchange information related to the condition. To subscribe, send an e-mail to: listserv@listserv.utoronto.ca

In the body of the message, type "subscribe PARKINSN," followed by your real name, for example: subscribe PARKINSN John Doe

Parkinson's Interaction Server/List/Forums
You'll find a caregivers' forum, an "Ask the Parkinson Dietitian" forum, a "Talk to a Speech Clinician" forum, and a public forum for patients and caregivers, all at the National Parkinson Foundation Web site. To sign up and participate in these forums, visit their Forums page.
http://www.Parkinson.org/shell/lyris.pl

CARE (Caregivers Are Really Essential) List
A list especially for caregivers of people with Parkinson's disease. A place to let off steam, express feelings, get practical support, and interact with other caregivers.
To subscribe, send an e-mail to:
listserv@listserv.muohio.edu
and in the body of the e-mail, type
subscribe CARE your full name

make sure you've turned off the "signature" feature in your e-mail when you send your subscribe request.

SPARKLE List
The SPARKLE list was created as an offshoot of the Parkinson's Disease Information Exchange Network. SPARKLE stands for "Smiling Parkies Live Easier." The SPARKLE list encourages jokes, Web sites, tributes, poems, riddles, chitchat, and friendship. You can find out more about the group and join the list at their Web site at: http://www.geocities.com/sparklelist
You can also join by sending a blank e-mail to:
join-sparkle@lyris.coles.org.uk

FREE PUBLICATIONS

National Parkinson Foundation Manuals

The National Parkinson Foundation publishes a variety of extremely helpful, free manuals. To order any of these free manuals, contact:

National Parkinson Foundation
1501 N.W. Ninth Avenue (Bob Hope Road)
Miami, FL 33136
(800) 327-4545

Parkinson's Disease: Fitness Counts
A 58-page manual from the National Parkinson Foundation, featuring exercises Parkinson's patients can do on their own at home.

Parkinson's Disease: Medications
A comprehensive 80-page booklet that features a listing of medications used by Parkinson's patients, including the medication, purpose, side effects, and other information.

Parkinson's Disease: Speaking Out
A 48-page manual detailing speech and voice problems, and techniques Parkinson's patients can use to help deal with these challenges.

Parkinson's Disease: Caring and Coping
A detailed 72-page guide for caregivers, offering practical information on providing assistance to Parkinson's patients, as well as self-care for caregivers.

Parkinson's Disease: Nutrition Matters
A 54-page manual discussing optimal nutrition for Parkinson's patients, constipation problems, and protein-balancing, including menus and recipes and other practical information.

Parkinson's Disease: What You and Your Family Should Know
A comprehensive 72-page guide providing an introduction and overview to Parkinson's, including information on diagnosis, treatment options, health maintenance, and other topics.

Publications from the National Parkinson Foundation, Orange County Chapter

Two free booklets are available from the National Parkinson Foundation, Orange County Chapter. The first booklet is titled *Dear Friends and Family* and was written from the point of view of a newly diagnosed Parkinson's patient. It features information for friends and family. *We Are There* is a guide for caregivers of Parkinson's patients that provides practical information on tasks such as cooking, assistance in the bathroom, dressing, speaking, exercise, and other topics. Single copies of each brochure can be sent by mail for free by contacting the National Parkinson Foundation, Orange County Chapter, 355 Placentia Avenue, #302, Newport Beach, CA 92663. Phone: 949-574-6338. Both booklets are also available in Acrobat (PDF) format, and can be downloaded free of charge on the Web at http://www.npfocc.org.

Free Parkinson's Disease Magazines

Parkinson's Disease Living Well

This is a helpful free quarterly magazine, published by several pharmaceutical companies. To subscribe, call toll-free (800) 371-1771.

Parkinson Report

A quarterly magazine, published by the National Parkinson Foundation, featuring detailed information for patients and practitioners. For information, call (800) 327-4545, except in Florida, call (800) 433-7022, and in California, call (800) 400-8488, or visit http://www.Parkinson.org on the Internet.

SELECTED WEB RESOURCES ON PARKINSON'S DISEASE

Dr. Jill's Parkinson's Site

Home page for this book, featuring links to key Web sites, updated information, and contact information for Dr. Jill Marjama-Lyons, coauthor of this book. The site also includes "Risks and Symptoms Checklist" to print and bring to the doctor, as well as a detailed Parkinson's disease glossary. http://www.DocJill.com

Wemove.org

A comprehensive resource for movement disorder information, which includes a uniquely detailed overview of the pharmacological and surgical treatments for Parkinson's disease. Also available are transcripts of past live chats with movement disorder specialists, plus a 24-hour live Parkinson's disease chat room for patients and caregivers.
http://www.wemove.org/

Parkinson's Information Exchange Network Online (P-I-E-N-O)

An excellent, comprehensive site, featuring a detailed and highly comprehensive drug database of hundreds of drugs Parkinson's patients may take, a variety of informational articles and resources, and support features.
http://www.parkinsons-information-exchange-network-online.com

Awakenings

An open forum, designed and written specifically for all with an interest in Parkinson's disease, including patients, their caregivers, primary care physicians, and specialists. This easy-to-navigate Web site is filled with reliable and helpful information, including tips on coping with the difficulties of day-to-day life.
http://www.parkinsonsdisease.com/

Rewired for Life

An online support group and informational resource for families and patients who have undergone or who are thinking about deep brain stimulation surgery to alleviate the symptoms of Parkinson's disease, essential tremor, intention tremor, and certain types of dystonia.
http://www.rewiredforlife.org/

Brain Talk Communities

Sponsored by the Department of Neurology at Massachusetts General Hospital, this site offers online patient support groups for a variety of neurological disorders, and features a very active bulletin board for Parkinson's disease.
http://neuro-mancer.mgh.harvard.edu/cgi-bin/Ultimate.cgi

Neurologychannel.com

A community monitored and developed by leading neurologists, this is an excellent resource for those seeking information on Parkinson's disease. This site provides valuable information on the symptoms, forms, and treatments of Parkinson's. Its special features include live patient-to-patient chats, bulletin boards, and a form that can help you find a neurologist in your area. You can also refer your questions directly to a board-certified neurologist during one of their live M.D. chats or at their Neurology Forum.

http://www.neurologychannel.com/parkinsonsdisease/index.shtml

Neurosurgery://on-call

This Web site, sponsored by the American Association of Neurological Surgeons and the Congress of Neurological Surgeons, contains a search engine to help you locate a board-certified neurosurgeon in your area. It also features an overview of Parkinson's disease, including an explanation of the medical and surgical treatments available.

http://www.neurosurgery.org/health/findaneurosurgeon.html

Parkinson's Disease, Living Well

A free online magazine, sponsored by two well-known pharmaceutical companies. This publication is "specifically designed to educate Parkinson's disease patients and their caregivers on the most up-to-date issues in Parkinson's disease management." At this site, you are able to view past issues and can request e-mail notification when the next issue becomes available.

http://www.parkinsonsweb.com/living_well/index.htm

People Living with Parkinson's

Established in 1999 by two women with early-onset PD, whose mission was to "create an atmosphere that encourages mutual support and friendship for people living with Parkinson's, their partners, family, and friends." This site contains chat rooms, forums, personal stories, links to PD information, and much more.

http://www.plwp.org/

PD Index: A Directory of Parkinson's Disease Information on the Internet

The personal home page of Phil Tompkins, who was diagnosed with Parkinson's disease in 1990. This easy-to-navigate Web site is filled with links to PD-related information, along with an article written by Mr. Tompkins entitled "Advice to the Newly Diagnosed."

http://www.pdindex.org

Young-Onset Parkinson's Disease

A personal home page written by a gentleman named Chris who was diagnosed with Parkinson's disease at the age of 35. The goals of his site are to highlight the "young-onset" aspects of Parkinson's disease and provide support to others by sharing his own thoughts and experiences.
http://www.young-parkinsons.org.uk/

WebMD's Parkinson's Center

Features news, a drug information database, diagnosis information, a support forum, a caregiver center, a free newsletter, and more.
http://my.webmd.com/condition_center/prk

James

An excellent British site about Parkinson's disease, featuring links, support information, and news. James also hosts a number of European mailing lists and other resources for European patients and families.
http://james.parkinsons.org.uk/index.html

Pallidotomy.com

The site of the Iacono Neuroscience Clinic, founded by Dr. Robert Iacono, M.D., F.A.C.S., features in-depth information on pallidotomy, including numerous patient testimonials, articles, and research summaries.
http://www.pallidotomy.com

The Center for Neurologic Study

A group of physicians at this nonprofit organization dedicated to research and treatment of neurological diseases have developed this Web site with the intent of sharing their current activities as a means of helping patients and families who have been affected by presently incurable neurologic disease. Click the "Publications" tab to find articles related to Parkinson's disease, including "Parkinson's Disease—Quality of Life Issues," and "The Parkinson Patient at Home."
http://www.cnsonline.org

Functional and Stereotactic Neurosurgery/Massachusetts General

This Web site from the Massachusetts General Hospital and Harvard Medical School provides clinical information regarding movement disorder surgeries. Although the articles are heavily laden with medical terminology, this site can be useful to families and patients seeking accurate information on surgery for Parkinson's disease.
http://neurosurgery.mgh.harvard.edu/fnctnlhp.htm

NYU Hospital for Joint Diseases' Comprehensive Center for Movement Disorders
This Web site, from the NYU Hospital for Joint Diseases' Comprehensive Center for Movement Disorders, provides detailed information on the various surgical treatments for Parkinson's disease, including deep brain stimulation (DBS), subthalamic nucleus (STN) deep brain stimulation, pallidotomy, and thalamotomy.
http://mcns10.med.nyu.edu/CMD/CMDmain.html

The Parkinson's Research Group
The Parkinson's Research Group, part of the world-renowned Mayo Clinic, is extremely interested in working with families who have two or more direct blood relatives with Parkinson's disease (or other movement disorders) in its quest to find out how much familial factors contribute to these conditions. In addition to outlining the group's current research, this site provides easy-to-understand information about Parkinson's disease for the patient, family, and caregiver.
http://www.mayo.edu/fpd/

The Parkinson's Recover Project
This site is "dedicated to dissemination of information regarding Parkinson's disease treatments which use techniques of Asian Medicine," and allows you to download a 222-page handbook that includes their theory, treatment, plans, and techniques for treating Parkinson's disease. (This handbook is intended as a guide for acupuncturists with training in Traditional Chinese Medicine or Five Element Theory, but is written in language that can be understood by those not in the field.)
http://www.pdtreatment.com/

The Parkinson's Disease Home Page at Holisticonline.com
Not only provides a basic overview of Parkinson's, but also compares modern Western medical treatments with alternative/integrative medical treatments for this disease. You'll find information on a variety of alternative treatments, including reflexology, acupuncture, and herbal remedies.
http://www.holisticonline.com/Remedies/Parkinson/pd_home.htm

Multimedia Healthcare Publications
Provides access to four geriatric-health-care–related journals, including *Clinical Geriatrics* and *Home Healthcare Consultant*. Search "Parkinson's"

and you will find a number of informative articles related to the emotional, physical, and quality-of-life issues associated with this disease.
http://www.mmhc.com/

Apples for Health

This innovative Web site offers up-to-date information on a variety of health-related issues. Search "Parkinson's disease" at Apples for Health and you'll receive a long list of unique and helpful articles. You can also subscribe to their weekly newsletter.
http://www.applesforhealth.com/index.html

Dr. Koop

This Web site is a good place to start for those seeking basic information about Parkinson's disease. Start by clicking the "Conditions" tab to answer such questions as "What is Parkinson's disease?" Then search the site to find more articles on various topics related to Parkinson's. You will also find information on complementary and alternative therapies by clicking on the "Natural Medicine" tab.
http://www.drkoop.com/

Healingwell.com's "Parkinson's Disease Library"

A user-friendly site that provides basic information on Parkinson's disease, plus informative feature articles such as "Ten Things Every Parkinson's Patient and Caregiver Should Know" and "The Healing Power of Physical Activity." Be sure to take "The Coping with Chronic Illness Self-Care Quiz" to gain insight on how well you are taking care of yourself.
http://www.healingwell.com/library/parkinsons/

Healthcentral.com

A large Web site offering information and products (including herbal recommendations) related to a variety of health conditions and diseases. Click "Parkinson's" in the "Conditions and Topics" box to find dozens of timely, newsworthy articles for the patient, family, and caregiver.
http://healthcentral.com

Infoaging.org

From the American Federation for Aging Research, an innovative Web site designed to provide the latest research on healthy aging. Search "Parkinson's" for up-to-date research-related articles. You can also subscribe to their newsletter to keep abreast of the recent news in the area of aging research. http://www.infoaging.org/index.html

Lycos Health with WebMD

Provides detailed information on Parkinson's disease, including causes, symptoms, and treatment. This site also addresses the diagnosis of "secondary parkinsonism," which is a disorder similar to Parkinson's disease, but caused by the effects of a medication or another disorder.
http://webmd.lycos.com/content/asset/adam_disease_shaking_palsy
http://webmd.lycos.com/content/asset/adam_disease_secondary_parkinsonism

American Academy of Family Physicians

This Web site, produced by the American Academy of Family Physicians, allows you to search the archives of their journal. Here you will find a copy of their patient information handout on Parkinson's disease, plus several informative articles related to the various clinical aspects of this disease.
http://www.aafp.org/afp/990415ap/2155.html

Intelihealth.com

One of the leading online health information sites provides easy-to-understand information to those seeking knowledge of Parkinson's disease. Use their search tool to find a number of related articles, and check out the archives of "Ask the Expert." This site is updated daily with headline medical news.
http://www.intelihealth.com

The National Institute of Environmental Health Sciences

Part of the National Institutes of Health, this organization is dedicated to reducing the burden of human illness and dysfunction from environmental causes. At their Web site, you will find information on past and present studies, which focus on the role environmental factors play in Parkinson's disease. Search "Parkinson's disease" for this and other noteworthy information.
http://www.niehs.nih.gov/

CBS Health Watch

From the people at Medscape, this is a user-friendly Web site filled with up-to-the-minute health-related news and articles. Search their library and

you'll find a comprehensive yet easy-to-understand article on the basic facts of Parkinson's disease, including information on "What Causes Parkinson's Disease" and "What Lifestyle Changes Can Help Parkinson's Disease."
http://www.cbshealthwatch.com

The Doctor Will See You Now
An innovative Web site filled with beneficial health and medical information. By using their search tool, you will find an overview of Parkinson's disease, including a thorough review of the medications used in treatment.
http://thedoctorwillseeyounow.com/

Senior Health at About.com
Offers a number of noteworthy links to Parkinson's disease Web sites. Click "Parkinson's disease" in the left-hand menu to find articles such as "Caregiver's Role" and "Nutritional Guidelines for Parkinson's Patients."
http://seniorhealth.about.com

Medscape
After registering at Medscape (a free and easy process), you will have access to one of the most highly respected medical search tools on the Internet. Search "Parkinson's disease" to find a multitude of links to articles, conference summaries, treatment updates, clinical management modules, practice guidelines, and textbooks.
http://www.medscape.com/

Medline Plus
A service of the National Library of Medicine, this is one of the definitive Internet resources for up-to-date, high-quality medical information. This site highlights the latest-breaking medical news and provides numerous links to informative articles and Web sites related to Parkinson's disease.
http://medlineplus.nlm.nih.gov/medlineplus/parkinsonsdisease.html

Postgraduate Medicine Online
This peer-reviewed journal for primary care physicians features the latest in clinical research translated into practical information. Although written for the practitioner, these archived articles offer a wealth of information to the patient and family. Simply use their search tool to locate PD-related articles.
http://www.postgradmed.com/back.htm

Classic Care Pharmacy

This Canadian site, from the pharmacists at Classic Care Pharmacy, provides a brief yet thorough overview of Parkinson's disease, including charts that detail the drugs that may cause parkinsonian features and the disorders that are sometimes mistaken for Parkinson's.

http://www.classiccare.on.ca/newsletter1.htm

Merck Manual of Diagnosis and Therapy

The Merck Manual of Diagnosis and Therapy, a highly trusted medical resource for over one hundred years, is now searchable on the Internet. This site provides a thorough explanation of Parkinson's disease, including detailed information on the drug therapies currently used.

http://www.merck.com/pubs/mmanual/section14/chapter179/179e.htm

Clinicaltrials.gov

Provides patients, family members, and members of the public current information regarding clinical research studies. This site, sponsored by NIH's U.S. National Library of Medicine, offers you the latest information on PD studies that are currently recruiting patients, including the purpose of the study, eligibility requirements, and contact information for those interested in participating.

http://clinicaltrials.gov/

Acurian Inc.

At Acurian.com, you are able to search for clinical trial listings related to Parkinson's disease (and other conditions), register to be considered for specific clinical trials, and keep abreast of advances in therapies and treatment options.

http://www.acurian.com/index.jsp

Centerwatch Clinical Trials Listing Service

An information source for the latest news and announcements from the clinical trials industry. Click "Patient and General Resources" to find links to the current trial listings of national and international research being conducted on a variety of diseases and conditions, including Parkinson's disease. In addition, you can request to be notified via e-mail about new trials in your area of interest, the results of clinical studies, and drugs recently approved by the FDA.

http://www.centerwatch.com/

Healthandage.com

Brought to you by the Novartis Foundation for Gerontology, the site focuses on gathering and sharing information on recent, practical, and cost-effective measures for health and disease management of older people. Use this site's search tool to find a variety of articles related to Parkinson's disease, including "Motivating Your Loved One With Parkinson's" and "Dealing with 'Wearing Off.'"
http://www.healthandage.com

The Family Caregiver Alliance

This site is one of the best Internet resources available to families who are caring for loved ones at home. Search "Parkinson's disease" to find a great variety of specialized information for the caregiver. You can also join fellow caregivers in conversation on topics such as coping mechanisms and safety strategies by subscribing to their online support group (e-mail format).
http://www.caregiver.org/

People of Life @ Home

This site offers a wide variety of home-modification products for elderly and handicapped persons living at home. Search this online store for items that can help you maintain a safe living environment for the Parkinson's patient. Or browse their archived articles for an interesting study of home-care–related issues, including "Parkinson's Disease: Effective Ways to Cope."
http://www.lifehome.com/Default.htm

Key to Care, "A Caregiver's Guide Through the Maze of Long-Term Care"

An invaluable resource for those who are caring for a loved one with Parkinson's disease. Here you will find a guide to understanding long-term care insurance, plus noteworthy information on living wills and health care proxies. There is also discussion on how to find a facility (be it adult day care, home care, or nursing home placement), and a Caregiver Support Discussion Forum.
http://www.keytocare.com/

Caregiver.com

Sponsored by Caregiver Media Group, a leading provider of information, support, and guidance for family and professional caregivers, this site en-

ables you to search for PD-related articles in the archives of *Today's Caregiver Magazine.*
http://www.caregiver.com/

National Family Caregivers Association (NFCA)

NFCA is "a grassroots organization created to educate, support, empower and speak up for the millions of Americans who care for chronically ill, aged or disabled loved ones." Caregivers will find tips on how to take charge of their lives, enabling them to have a higher quality of life and to make a positive contribution to the care recipient's well-being.
http://www.nfcacares.org/

MEDITOPIA

This alternative-medicine site explores Parkinson's disease from a Traditional Oriental Medicine (TOM) point of view.
http://meditopia.com/dis/park/otpark.html

Healthphone.com

Founded by a group of scientists and Chinese and natural medical practitioners, this site is devoted to "demystifying and promoting the arts of Chinese and natural medicines to the world." Click "Consumer Site" on their home page and then highlight "Parkinson's disease" in their list of 130 ailments to learn about Traditional Chinese Medicine's detailed treatment plan for this disease. Includes information on acupuncture, moxibustion, Qi Gong, acupressure, shiatsu, and more.
http://www.healthphone.com

OmAge.com

The New Age healers at OmAge.com have outlined an alternative medical approach to the treatment of Parkinson's disease. On this page you will find details of their holistic plan of care, including elements of aromatherapy, homeopathic treatment, color and sound reflexology, and pranic healing.
http://www.omage.com/january/people/qa.htm

The Natural Pharmacist

Provides extensive information on natural health treatments for a multitude of medical conditions, including Parkinson's disease. This site can also answer your questions regarding which herbs and nutrients might be harmful (or helpful) if combined with your medications.
http://www.thenaturalpharmacist.com

Meridian Institute
This nonprofit organization, dedicated to researching holistic and integrative approaches to wellness and healing, provides the results of their research study, which explored the effectiveness of the Edgar Cayce treatment recommendations for Parkinson's disease. A bulletin board is available to post questions to members of the institute.
http://www.meridianinstitute.com

Natural Healthsite.com
Offers holistic protocols for living with Parkinson's disease, which include vitamins/minerals/supplements, botanicals, homeopathic remedies, and more.
http://www.naturalhealthsite.com/Parkins.htm

BOOKS ON PARKINSON'S DISEASE

The following books on Parkinson's disease may also be a help to you in your quest to understand and learn more about this condition.

Lucky Man: A Memoir
by Michael J. Fox
Hyperion, 2002

Understanding Parkinson's Disease: A Self-Help Guide
by David L. Cram, M.D.
LPC, 1999

Parkinson's Disease—Questions and Answers, 3rd ed.
by Robert A. Hauser et al.
Merit Publishing International, 2000

When Parkinson's Strikes Early: Voices, Choices, Resources, and Treatment
by Barbara Blake-Krebs, M.A., et al.
Hunter House 2001

Parkinson's Disease: A Complete Guide for Patients and Families
by William J. Weiner, M.D., et al.
Johns Hopkins Press Health Book 2001

Parkinson's Disease and the Art of Moving
by John Argue
New Harbinger Publications, 2000

Caring for the Parkinson Patient: A Practical Guide
by J. Thomas Hutton (editor) et al.
Prometheus Books, 1999

Shaking Up Parkinson
by Abraham Lieberman, M.D.
Jones & Bartlett Publishers, 2001

Preventing Falls: A Defensive Approach
by J. Thomas Hutton, M.D., Ph.D. (editor), et al.
Prometheus Books, 2000

Eat Well, Stay Well with Parkinson's Disease
By Kathrynne Holden, M.S., R.D.
Five Star Living, 1998

Brain Recovery: Powerful Therapy for Challenging Brain Disorders
by David Perlmutter, M.D.
Perlmutter, 2000
http://www.brainrecovery.com

EXERCISE

Parkinson's Disease: Fitness Counts
A free, 58-page manual from the National Parkinson Foundation, featuring exercises Parkinson's patients can do on their own at home. To obtain a copy, contact:

National Parkinson Foundation
1501 N.W. Ninth Avenue (Bob Hope Road)
Miami, FL 33136
(800) 327-4545

Parkinson's Disease and the Art of Moving
by John Argue
New Harbinger, 2000

This 220-page book features exercises derived from yoga and t'ai chi, helping Parkinson's patients cope with loss of coordination and relearn how to sit up, get up from a sitting position, speak clearly, keep balance, and other important functions.
http://www.parkinsonsexercise.com

Jodi Stolove's Chair Dancing
An aerobic workout program, presented on video or audiocassette, that is designed to be performed in a chair.

http://www.chairdancing.com
(800) 551-4FUN

NATIONAL PARKINSON FOUNDATION CENTERS OF EXCELLENCE

Arizona

Muhammad Ali Parkinson Research Center
Barrow Neurological Institute
St. Joseph's Hospital and Medical Center
500 West Thomas Road, Suite 720
Phoenix, AZ 85013
(602) 406-4931
http://www.thebni.com/lrngcntr.asp?=lc_park&supnav=lc_park_supnav
maprc@chw.edu

California

Hoag Hospital
355 Placentia, Suite 302
Newport Beach, CA 92658-6100
(949) 574-6338

The Parkinson's Institute
1170 Morse Avenue
Sunnyvale, CA 94089
(408) 734-2800 Ext. 644

The Parkinson's Center at St. John's
1600 North Rose Avenue
Oxnard, CA 93030
(805) 988-2500 x2004
http://www.stjohnshealth.org/index.asp?catID=ps&pg=ps_parkinson

University of California, San Diego
The Salk Institute
9500 Gilman Drive
San Diego, CA 92093-0948
(619) 622-5800

University of California, San Francisco
Parkinson Disease Clinic
503 Parnassas Street, Room M348
San Francisco, CA 94143-0216
(415) 476-9276
http://www.sf.med.va.gov/research/pd/surgery.htm

University of Southern California Los Angeles
NPF Clinic/Department of Neurology
1510 San Pablo Street, HCC Suite 268
Los Angeles, CA 90033-4606
(323) 442-5791
http://www.parkinsons-usc.org/

Colorado

Colorado Neurological Institute
701 East Hampden Avenue, Suite 530
Englewood, CO 80110-2776
(303) 788-4600
http://www.TheCNI.org

Florida

NPF Care Center Shands—Jacksonville
580 West Eighth Street, 9th Floor
Jacksonville, FL 32209

(904) 244-9818
http://www.Parkinson.org/npfcc.htm

NPF Care Center Tallahassee Memorial
NeuroScience Center
1213 Hodges Drive
Tallahassee, FL 32308
(850) 681-5082
http://www.Parkinson.org/npfcc.htm

NPF Care Center Fort Lauderdale
North Ridge Medical Center
5757 N. Dixie Highway, Room 122
Ft. Lauderdale, FL 33334
(954) 202-1274
http://www.Parkinson.org/npfcc.htm

NPF Care Center Orlando
Orlando Regional Healthcare
1404 Kuhl Avenue, 3rd floor
Orlando, FL 32806
(407) 841-5111 Ext. 1319

NPF Care Center West Palm Beach
St. Mary's Medical
901 45th Street
West Palm Beach, FL 33407
(561) 882-9137
http://www.Parkinson.org/npfcc.htm

Parkinson Association of Southwest Florida
P.O. Box 9778
Naples, FL 34101
(941) 591-2006
http://www.pasfi.org
Pasfi@aol.com

Parkinson Center of Excellence
Neurological Associates
1888 Hillview Street

Sarasota, FL 34258
(941) 366-5880
http://www.neuro-fl.com

University of Florida College of Medicine
109 Grinter Hall
Box 100236, UFHSC
Gainesville, FL 31610-0236
(352) 392-3491

University of Miami
Department of Neurology
1501 N.W. Ninth Avenue
Miami, FL 33136
(305) 547-6327

University of South Florida Movement Disorder Center
Harbourside Medical Tower, Suite 410
Tampa, FL 33602
(813) 253-4455
http://hsc.usf.edu/NEURO/usf.html

Hawaii

Kuakini Medical Center
347 North Kuakini Street, HPM-9
Honolulu, HI 96817
(808) 523-8461
http://www.parkinson.org/groups/kuakini.htm

Illinois

Southern Illinois University School of Medicine
Department of Neurology
P.O. Box 19643
Springfield, IL 62794-9643
(217) 524-7879
http://www.siumed.edu/neuro/

Neurologic Associates, Inc.
11824 Southwest Highway
Palo Heights, IL 60463-1055

University of Illinois at Chicago
Department of Neurology, M/C 796
Neuropsychiatric Institute
912 South Wood Street, Room 855N
Chicago, IL 60612-7330
(312) 413-9680
http://www.uic.edu/depts/mcne/Parkinson

Kansas

University of Kansas Neurological Center
3901 Rainbow Boulevard
Kansas City, KS 66160
(913) 588-6970
http://www.kumc.edu/parkinson/

Maryland

National Institute of Neurological Disorders and Stroke (NINDS)
National Institutes of Health (NIH)
Building 10, Room 5C106
10 Center Drive, MSC 1406
Bethesda, MD 20892-1406
(301) 496-4604
http://www.ninds.nih.gov/

Massachusetts

Massachusetts General Hospital
A Harvard Medical School Affiliate
VBK 915
55 Fruit Street
Boston, MA 02114
(617) 726-5532
(617) 726-2000 (hospital switchboard)
(617) 726-8581 for national and international referrals

(617) 277-2381 for local emergency neurosurgical hotline
http://neurosurgery.mgh.harvard.edu/fnctnlhp.htm

Michigan

Sinai Hospital
Clinical Neuroscience Center
26400 West Twelve Mile Road, Suite 110
Southfield, MI 48034
(248) 355-3875

Minnesota

Struther's Parkinson Center
6701 Country Club Drive
Golden Valley, MN 55427
(612) 993-5495
http://www.methodisthospital.com/struthersparkinsons/

Nevada

Sunrise Hospital
3131 La Canada, Suite 107
Las Vegas, NV 89109
(702) 731-8329

New York

Beth Israel Medical Center
10 Union Square East, Suite 2R
New York, NY 10003
(212) 844-8482
http://www.parkinsonsdiseaseny.org

Kings County Hospital and SUNY
450 Clarkson Avenue, Box 1213
Brooklyn, NY 11203
(212) 982-5850

The Mount Sinai Medical Center
One Gustave L. Levy Place
New York, NY 10029
(212) 241-2869
http://www.mssm.edu/neurology/research.html

North Shore University Hospital
Movement Disorders Center
444 Community Drive
Manhasset, NY 11030
(516) 562-2498

University of Rochester
Medical Center
601 Elmwood Avenue, Box 673
Rochester, NY 14642
(716) 275-1274

Ohio

Ohio State University
Medical Center
1581 McCampbell Hall, Suite 371
Columbus, OH 43210-1128
(614) 688-4056
http://www.parkinson-ohiostate.org/

Oregon

Oregon Health Sciences University
3181 S.W. Sam Jackson Park Road, L226
Box 494
Portland, OR 97201-3098
(503) 494-5620
http://www.ohsu.edu/som-neuro/parkinsons/

Pennsylvania

Parkinson's Disease and Movement Disorders Center at Pennsylvania Hospital
330 South Ninth Street, 3rd floor
Philadelphia, PA 19107
(215) 829-7273
http://www.pahosp.com/services/bdy5j3.htm

University of Pittsburgh
540 Crawford Hall
Pittsburgh, PA 15260
(412) 692-4610

Tennessee

Vanderbilt University
1601 23rd Avenue South, Suite 313
Nashville, TN 37212
(615) 327-7080
http://www.mc.vanderbilt.edu/neurology/Move.htm

Texas

Baylor College of Medicine
6550 Fannin, Suite 1801
Houston, TX 77030-3498
(713) 798-3951
http://www.bcm.tmc.edu/neurol/struct/park/park1.html
neurons@bcm.tmc.edu

Neurology Research and Education Center at Covenant Health System
4102 24th Street, Suite 501
Lubbock, TX 79410
(806) 796-2647
http://neuroresearch.com

Scott & White Clinic
Texas A&M University Health Science Center

College of Medicine
2401 South 31 Street
Temple, TX 76508

University of Texas Southwestern Medical Center
5323 Harry Hines Boulevard
Dallas, TX 75235-8897

Washington

Parkinson Education Society of Puget Sound
Park Rose Care Center
3919 South Nineteenth
Tacoma, WA 98405
(253) 752-5677

Wisconsin

Sinai-Samaritan Medical Center/The Wisconsin
Parkinson's Association
3070 North 51st Street, Suite 206
Milwaukee, WI 53210-1688
(414) 871-6988
http://www.parkcntr.org

OTHER NOTABLE PARKINSON'S DISEASE RESOURCES

Columbia Presbyterian Medical Center—Center for Parkinson Disease
and Other Movement Disorders
622 W. 168th Street
New York, NY 10032
(212) 305-2500
http://cpmcnet.columbia.edu

Glenbrook and Evanston Hospitals—Pallidotomy Program
Glenbrook: 2100 Pfingsten Road, Glenview, IL 60025
Evanston: 2650 Ridge Avenue, Evanston, IL 60201
(847) 657-1691
http://pubweb.acns.nwu.edu/~mre970/pallidot.htm

Henry Ford Hospital
One Ford Place
Detroit, MI 48202
(313) 876-2600 (switchboard)
Toll-free (800) 653-6568 (appointments)
http://www.henryfordhealth.org

North Shore University Hospital
300 Community Drive
Manhasset, NY 11030
(516) 562-0100

Perlmutter Health Center
720 Goodlette Road North, #203
Naples, FL 34102
(941) 649-7400
http://www.perlhealth.com

Wake Forest University Baptist Medical Center
Medical Center Boulevard
Winston-Salem, NC 27157
(336) 716-2011
http://www.bgsm/edu/bgsm/surg-sci/ns/pd.html

ADAPTIVE CLOTHING AND ASSISTIVE DEVICES

For easy-on and accessible clothing, and other assistive devices, here are some companies and Web sites to investigate:

Finally It Fits
100-A Gilman Avenue
Campbell, CA 95008
(408) 866-9805
http://www.finallyitfits.net

Accessible Threads
1218 Central Street
Evanston, IL 80201
(847) 475-7078
http://www.accessiblethreads.com

Clothing/Assistive Devices List
http://www.planetamber.com/resources/198.html

Adaptive Clothing—Web Sites List
http://www.kansas.net/~cbaslock/chothint.html

SERVICE DOGS

Independence Dogs: Service Dogs for the Mobility Impaired
146 State Line Road
Chadds Ford, PA 19317
http://www.independencedogs.org
(610) 358-2723

DIETARY, NUTRITIONAL, AND HERBAL MEDICINE APPROACHES

Barbara Maddoux, R.N., D.O.M.
ClearHealth
7510 Montgomery Boulevard, N.E., Suite 202
Albuquerque, NM 87109
(505) 884-4646
http://www.clearhealth.com
btyoga@aol.com

Barbara Maddoux is a licensed nurse, a board-certified acupuncturist and Chinese herbologist, clinical nutritionist, Doctor of Oriental Medicine, and student and teacher of yoga. She runs ClearHealth, an Albuquerque-based practice that specializes in integrating Chinese medicine, acupuncture, herbology, and nutrition—plus a functional medicine approach to health assessment—for optimal wellness.

Wanda Barnes, R.N.
Certified Kripalu Yoga Instructor
Jacksonville, Florida area
E-mail: WandaBar@msn.com

The One Earth Herbal Sourcebook: Everything You Need to Know about Chinese, Western, and Ayurvedic Herbal Treatments
by Alan Keith Tillotson, Ph.D., A.H.G., D.Ay., with Nai-shing Hu Tillotson, O.M.D., L.Ac., and Robert Abel, Jr., M.D.
Kensington Publishing, 2001

The definitive, comprehensive guide about herbal medicine. A must-have manual for anyone interested in nutritional approaches and supplements, from one of the nation's premier herbalists.

Herbal Defense: Positioning Yourself to Triumph over Illness and Aging
by Robyn Landis, with Karta Purkh Singh Khalsa
Warner Books, 1997

An excellent guide to use of herbal medicine to prevent or treat specific illnesses, from another of the nation's most respected herbalists.

Prescription for Natural Healing
by James F. Balch, M.D., and Phyllis A. Balch.
Avery Penguin Putnam, 2000

A comprehensive reference featuring nutritional supplements, vitamins, and recommendations.

Dr. Atkins' Vita-Nutrient Solution: Nature's Answers to Drugs
by Robert D. Atkins, M.D.
Simon & Schuster, 1998

Excellent overview, with specific recommendations regarding supplements—including dosages—for different autoimmune conditions and other health issues.

American Herbalists Guild
Herbalist Referral page:
http://www.americanherbalist.com/referral_search.htm

Enter your state in the search box and hit "Submit," and you'll see AHG herbalists in your area. You can call (770) 751-6021.

Herb Research Foundation
1007 Pearl Street, Suite 200
Boulder, CO 80302
(800) 748-2617

Herbal Hotline: (303) 449-2265
http://www.herbs.org

Information on herbal support specifically for particular conditions is available in a detailed packet. They also have a specialized Herbal Hotline to answer specific questions, for a small fee.

American Dietetic Association's Nationwide Nutrition Network
(800) 366-1655
Database: http://www.eatright.org/finddiet.html

This organization offers referrals to registered dietitians, and a searchable online database of registered dietitians.

Nutrition Web Site
http://nutrition.about.com

Rick Hall's excellent site provides a comprehensive Web-based starting point for nutritional information.

American Association of Naturopathic Physicians
2366 Eastlake Avenue East, Suite 322
Seattle, WA 98102
(206) 323-7610
Referral line: (206) 298-0125
Web site database: http://www.naturopathic.org/find_nd.htm

This group offers a referral line, directory, and brochures explaining naturopathic medicine.

American Holistic Health Association
Department R
P.O. Box 17400
Anaheim, CA 92817-7400
(714) 779-6152
http://ahha.org

A nonprofit organization with various self-help resources, free booklets, and other information available by mail or on the Web.

National Center for Homeopathy
801 N. Fairfax Street, Suite 306
Alexandria, VA 22314

(703) 548-7790
http://www.healthworld.com/nch

Provides information on homeopathy, and referrals to qualified practitioners in your area.

Great Smokies Diagnostic Laboratory
63 Zillicoa Street
Asheville, NC 28801
(800) 522-4762
http://www.gsdl.com
cs@gsdl.com

The nation's top lab for functional medicine testing.

Books about Diet/Nutrition

Eat Well, Stay Well with Parkinson's Disease
by Kathrynne Holden, M.S., R.D.
Five Star Living, 1998

The Glucose Revolution: The Authoritative Guide to the Glycemic Index—The Groundbreaking Medical Discovery
by Thomas M. S. Wolever, M.D., Ph.D., Jennie Brand-Miller, Ph.D. (editor), Kaye Foster-Powell, and Stephen Colagiuri, M.D.
Marlow & Co., 1999

The Good Carb Cookbook : Secrets of Eating Low on the Glycemic Index
by Sandra Woodruff
Avery Penguin Putnam, 2001

CHINESE MEDICINE/ACUPUNCTURE

National Certification Commission for Acupuncture and Oriental Medicine (NCCAOM)
11 Canal Center Plaza, Suite 300
Alexandria, VA 22314
(703) 548-9004
http://www.nccaom.org

The NCCAOM awards the title Dipl.Ac. to acupuncture practitioners who pass its certification requirements. You can get a list of Diplomates of Acupuncture in your state from them for $3.

American Association of Oriental Medicine
433 Front Street
Catasauqua, PA 18032
(888) 500-7999
http://www.aaom.org

AAOM provides referrals to practitioners who are state-licensed or certified by various respected certifying organizations. They also have an online state-by-state referral search for TCM and acupuncture practitioners at http://www.aaom.org/referral.html.

American Academy of Medical Acupuncture
(800) 521-2262

The AAMA, which provides referrals, requires that its members (who are all physicians) undergo at least 220 hours of continuing medical education in acupuncture.

Accreditation Commission for Acupuncture and Oriental Medicine
(301) 608-9680

This organization can verify which American schools of acupuncture and Oriental medicine have a decent reputation.

American Foundation of Traditional Chinese Medicine
505 Beach Street
San Francisco, CA 94133
(415) 776-0503

This organization provides information on Traditional Chinese Medicine, as well as practitioner referrals.

National Acupuncture and Oriental Medicine Alliance
14637 Starr Road S.E.
Olalla, WA 98359
Phone: (253) 851-6896
Fax: (253) 851-6883

Professional organization that represents licensed, registered, or certified acupuncture and Oriental medicine practitioners. They provide practitioner referrals.

Dr. Patrick Purdue's Web Site
http://www.PatrickPurdue.com

Excellent Web site featuring information from this renowned Traditional Chinese Medicine practitioner.

Acupuncture.com
http://www.acupuncture.com/Referrals/ref2.htm

Acupuncture.com offers a list of licensed acupuncturists by state.

TRADITIONAL MENTAL HEALTH SUPPORT

For traditional mental health support, such as a psychologist, a counselor, or general support groups, contact:

National Mental Health Association
1021 Prince Street
Alexandria, VA 22314-2971
(800) 969-NMHA

Provides referrals to state and regional mental health associations and resources.

National Mental Health Consumers Self-Help Clearinghouse
1211 Chestnut Street, Suite 1000
Philadelphia, PA 19107
(800) 553-4539
info@mhselfhelp.org

Offers articles and books on consumer-oriented and mental health issues, and a reference file on relevant groups, organizations, and agencies.

Mental Health Site
http://mentalhealth.about.com.

Dr. Leonard Holmes's comprehensive site on mental health.

INTRAVENOUS GLUTATHIONE THERAPY

David Perlmutter, M.D.
Perlmutter Health Center
Commons Medical Center
800 Goodlette Road North, Suite 270
Naples, FL 34102
(800) 530-1982 or (941) 649-7400
http://www.perlhealth.com
http://www.brainrecovery.com
info@brainrecovery.com

Dr. Perlmutter is willing to speak with other doctors if they're interested in investigating the glutathione therapy.

Wellness Pharmacy
For IV glutathione by prescription mail order, and a list of doctors who are using the therapy.
(800) 227-2627
http://www.wellnesshealth.com

Glutathione Therapy in Parkinson's Disease
An informational/instructional video from David Perlmutter, M.D.
(800) 530-1982

SPIRITUALITY AND HEALTH

George Washington Institute for Spirituality and Health
George Washington University Medical Center
Warwick Building, Room 336
2300 K Street, N.W.
Washington, DC 20037
(202) 994-0971
http://www.gwish.org

Excellent organization pioneering integration of spirituality into medical education and practice.

MIND-BODY SUPPORT

Stress Reduction
http://stress.about.com.
Melissa Stöppler, M.D.'s excellent site on stress reduction

Mind Body Medical Institute
http://www.mbmi.org
110 Francis Street
Boston, MA 02215
(617) 632-9530

Herbert Benson, M.D.'s Harvard-based organization that has pioneered the study and practice of mind-body medicine.

The Center for Mind/Body Medicine
P.O. Box 1048
La Jolla, CA 92038
(619) 794-2425

Developed under the guidance of Deepak Chopra, M.D., this organization offers both residential and outpatient programs, as well as education and training programs in Ayurveda.

American Chronic Pain Association
P.O. Box 850
Rocklin, CA 95677
(916) 632-0922

This group manages a list of over five hundred support groups internationally and publishes workbooks and a newsletter.

Center for Attitudinal Healing
33 Buchanan
Sausalito, CA 94965
(415) 331-6161

Support groups throughout the nation for people with chronic or serious illness.

Wellness Community
2716 Ocean Park Boulevard, Suite 1040

Santa Monica, CA 90405
(310) 314-2555

Chapters throughout the nation offer support groups for people with chronic or serious illness.

REIKI

Holistic Healing Site and Spiral Visions
http://healing.about.com
http://www.spiralvisions.com

Web sites of Usui Reiki Master Phylameana lila Desy, offering comprehensive Reiki information, articles, community, and links.

Essential Reiki: A Complete Guide to an Ancient Healing Art
by Diane Stein
Crossing Press, 1995

A definitive book introducing Reiki and providing an overview of this healing art.

PATIENT EMPOWERMENT

Marie Savard, M.D., and DrSavard.com
Marie Savard, M.D., is an internationally known internist, women's health expert, and patients' rights champion. She is author of two essential books for all patients: *How to Save Your Own Life: The Savard System for Managing—and Controlling—Your Health Care,* which is a helpful guide to medical tests, procedures, and effectively working with doctors on your own behalf, and *The Savard Health Record,* a binder-format workbook that organizes all your critical health information in one location. Dr. Savard's Web site, http://www.drsavard.com, has free online downloadable office visit forms and health-at-a-glance forms for organizing your own health information.
Marie Savard, M.D.
Savard Systems
54 Churchill Drive
York, PA 17403

(877) SAVARDS (728-2737)
http://www.drsavard.com

Your Doctor in the Family.com
http://YourDoctorintheFamily.com

Richard Fogoros, M.D., has developed an excellent site that empowers patients and provides helpful information.

HOLISTIC/COMPLEMENTARY/ALTERNATIVE PRACTITIONERS

American Osteopathic Association
142 East Ontario Street
Chicago, IL 60611
(800) 621-1773
www@aoa.nat.org
http://www.aoa-net.org

The American Osteopathic Association has state referral lists for osteopaths in all fifty states.

American Board of Medical Specialties "Certified Doctor" Service
(800) 776-2378
http://www.abms.org

This is an online service that allows you to browse for doctors by specialty and locale and get certification information on specific docs. These are conventional doctors.

American Medical Association (AMA) "Physician Select"
http://www.amaassn.org/aps/amahg.htm

The AMA's Physician Select program allows you to browse their database for AMA member doctors, almost always conventional doctors. It lists medical school and year graduated, residency training, primary practice, secondary practice, major professional activity, and board certification for all doctors who are licensed physicians.

American Holistic Health Association
P.O. Box 17400
Anaheim, CA 92817-7400
(714) 779-6152

http://www.ahha.org/
ahha@healthy.net

The American Holistic Health Association offers an online referral to its members, who are holistic doctors.

American Holistic Medical Association
6728 Old McLean Village Drive
McLean, VA 22101
(703) 556-9728
Patient Information number: (703) 556-9728
http://www.holisticmedicine.org
info@holisticmedicine.org

The American Holistic Medical Association publishes a Referral Directory of member M.D.s and D.O.s.

GENERAL DOCTOR REFERRAL SERVICES

American Board of Medical Specialties
1007 Church Street, Suite 404
Evanston, IL 60201-5913
Main number: (847) 491-9091
Phone Verification of Doctors and their Specialties:
(866) ASK-ABMS
Online search: http://www.abms.org/newsearch.asp

Hospital Referrals
If a good hospital in your area has a referral service, this can be a decent source of information on and referrals to doctors. If the hospital's reputation is good, the doctors typically are going to be of a better caliber. Some of the more sophisticated hospital referral services will offer educational and practice-style information about doctors in their databases.

U.S. News and World Report's "Best Graduate Schools"/Medical School Evaluation
(800) 836-6397
http://www.usnews.com/usnews/edu/beyond/gradrank/med/gdmedt1.htm

You can evaluate whether or not your doctor went to a good medical school by checking the med school rankings provided by *U.S. News and World Re-*

port. The information is available on the Web. You can also order their "Best Graduate Schools" directory, for $5.95, at the Web site, or by calling their 800 number.

Doctor Ratings

Find out if any of your local magazines rate doctors. *Washingtonian* magazine, for example, periodically asks doctors to pick those other Washington, D.C./Maryland/Virginia–area doctors they'd most recommend in particular specialties, and publishes the results. It's always a comfort to me to see a doctor I've been referred to appear on this list, although it doesn't always guarantee I'll *like* that doctor!

Best Doctors
(888) DOCTORS
http://www.bestdoctors.com

Best Doctors has a "Family Doc Finder" at their Web site, where, for a small fee, you can find recommended primary care physicians in your area. You'll find only conventional doctors via this service. Best Doctors also conducts specialized physician searches for rare, catastrophic, or serious illnesses. The specialized search, which costs $1,500, is merited only in the direst situations, but it's worth knowing about if you find yourself seriously in need of a specialist or expert.

CHECKING OUT BAD DOCTORS

Questionable Doctors Listing
(202) 588-1000
http://www.questionabledoctors.org

Check on whether your doctor has been listed in the *16,638 Questionable Doctors* report, which was produced by the consumer advocacy group Public Citizen. The book, also available in CD form, lists more than twenty thousand doctors who were disciplined by state medical boards or federal agencies. Among these doctors were those accused of sexual abuse, substandard care, incompetence or negligence, criminal conviction, misprescribing drugs, and substance abuse. Interestingly, up to 69 percent of these doctors are still practicing medicine.

Medical Board Charges or Actions
You can find out whether disciplinary action has ever been taken with your doctor, or whether charges are pending against him or her, by calling your state medical board. A good list of all medical boards is found at http://www.fsmb.org/members.htm. You can also search at the Association of State Medical Board Executive Directors' "DocFinder" service, http://www.docboard.org/.

INCONTINENCE RESOURCES AND SUPPORT

National Association for Continence
P.O. Box 8306
Spartanburg, SC 29305-8306
(800) BLADDER ([800] 252-3337)

Simon Foundation for Continence
P.O. Box 835
Wilmette, IL 60091
(800) 237-4666

National Kidney and Urologic Diseases Information Clearinghouse
3 Information Way
Bethesda, MD 20892-3580

SLEEP DIFFICULTIES RESOURCES AND SUPPORT

American Sleep Apnea Association
1424 K Street N.W., Suite 302
Washington, DC 20005
(202) 293-3650
http://www.sleepapnea.org
asaa@sleepapnea.org

Better Sleep Council
501 Wythe Street
Alexandria, VA 22314
(703) 683-8371
http://www.bettersleep.org

Narcolepsy Network
10921 Reed Hartman Highway, Suite 119
Cincinnati, OH 45242
(513) 891-3522
http://www.narcolepsynetwork.org

National Center for Sleep Disorders Research
6701 Rockledge Drive, MSC 7920
Bethesda, MD 20892-7920
(301) 435-0199
http://www.nhlbi.nih.gov/health/public/sleep

National Sleep Foundation
1522 K Street, N.W., Suite 500
Washington, DC 20005-1253
(202) 347-3471
http://www.sleepfoundation.org

Restless Legs Syndrome Foundation
819 Second Street S.W.
Rochester, MN 55902-2985
(507) 287-6465
http://www.rls.org
rlsfoundation@rls.org

DEPRESSION RESOURCES AND SUPPORT

**The National Institute of Mental Health's (NIMH) Depression
Awareness, Recognition, and Treatment Program**
Information Resources and Inquiries Branch
Room 7C-02, MSC 8030
Bethesda, MD 20892-8030
(800) 421-4211
http://www.nimh.nih.gov.

(Note: Ask for a copy of their publication *If You're Over 65 and Feeling Depressed: Treatment Brings New Hope.*)

National Depressive and Manic Depressive Association (National DMDA)
730 N. Franklin Street, Suite 501
Chicago, IL 60610-3526
(800) 826-3632
http://www.ndmda.org

This organization has two hundred chapters in the United States and Canada offering support to people with depression and their families. It sponsors education and research programs and distributes brochures, videotapes, and audio programs.

National Alliance for the Mentally Ill (NAMI)
200 North Glebe Road, Suite 1015
Arlington, VA 22203-3754
(800) 950-NAMI (6264)
http://www.nami.org

NAMI offers a Medical Information Series that provides patients and families with information on several mental illnesses and their treatments, including the publication "Understanding Major Depression: What You Need to Know about This Medical Illness." NAMI state affiliates provide emotional support and can help find local services.

National Mental Health Association (NMHA)
1021 Prince Street
Alexandria, VA 22314-2971
(800) 969-6642
http://www.nmha.org

Publishes information on a variety of mental health issues and has special information on depression and its treatment. NMHA also provides referrals and support.

American Association for Geriatric Psychiatry (AAGP)
7910 Woodmont Avenue, Suite 1350
Bethesda, MD 20814-3004
http://www.aagpgpa.org

A national professional organization of specialists in geriatric psychiatry. It provides teaching materials and brochures about selected mental health disorders, including depression.

Appendix B
References

Chapter 1

Fahn, S., Elton, R., and members of the UPDRS Developmental Committee. "Unified Parkinson's Disease Rating Scale." *Recent Developments in Parkinson's Disease,* vol. 2. Florham Park, N.J.: Macmillan, 1987, pp. 153–163, 293–304.

Flaherty, A. W., and Graybiel, A. M. "Anatomy of the Basal Ganglia." *Movement Disorders* vol. 3. Oxford: Butterworth-Heinemann, 1994, p. 3.

Hoehn, M. M., and Yahr, M. D. "Parkinsonism: Onset, progression and mortality." *Neurology* 1967; 17:427–442.

Koller, W. C., Silver, D. E., and Lieberman, A. "An algorithm for the management of Parkinson's disease." *Neurology* 1994; 44(10):1.

Marsden, S., et. al., *Movement Disorders,* vol. 3. Oxford: Butterworth-Heinemann, 1994, p. 3.

Martilla, R. J., and Rinne, U. K. "Epidemiological approaches to the etiology of Parkinson's disease." *Act Neurol Scand* 1989; 126:13–18.

Martilla, R. J., and Rinne, U. K. "Epidemiology of Parkinson's disease in Finland." *Act Neurol Scand* 1976; 53(2):81–102.

Parkinson J. *An Essay on the Shaking Palsy.* London: Whittingham and Rowland for Sherwood, Neely and Jones, 1817.

Shultz, Kennedy J. *You Are the Power: A Guide to Personal Greatness.* Carlsbad, CA: Hay House, Inc., 1993.

Chapter 2

Baldereschi, M., et al. "Parkinson's disease and parkinsonism in a longitudinal study. Two-fold higher incidence in men." *Neurology* 2000; 55:1358–1363.

Benedetti, M. D., et al. "Hysterectomy, menopause and estrogen preceding Parkinson's disease: An exploratory case-controlled study." *Mov Disor* 2001; 16:830–837.

Benedetti, M. D., et al. "Smoking, alcohol and coffee consumption preceding Parkinson's disease: A case-control study." *Neurology* 2000; 55:1350–1358.

Bertarbet, R., et al. "Chronic systemic pesticide exposure reproduces features of Parkinson's disease." *Nat Neurosci* 2000; 3(12):1301–1306.

Duvoisin, R. "Role of genetics in the cause of Parkinson's disease." *Mov Disor* 1998; 13:7–12.

Gil, S. S., et al. "Intraparenchymal putaminal administration of glial-derived neurotrophic factor in the treatment of advanced Parkinson's disease," Reports from the 54th Annual Meeting of the American Academy of Neurology, April 13–20, 2002. *Neurology* 2002; 58 (supplement 7).

Goetz, C. G. *Neurotoxins in Clinical Practice.* New York: SP Medical and Scientific, 1985, p xix.

Golbe, L. I., Farrell, T. M., and Davis, P. H. "Case-control study of early life dietary factors in Parkinson's disease." *Arch Neurol* 1988; 45:350–353.

Golbe, L. I., et al. "A large kindred with Parkinson's disease." *Ann Neurol* 1990; 27:276–282.

Golbe, L. I., Lazzarini A. M., Schwartz, K. O., et al. "Autosomal dominant parkinsonism with benign course and typical Lewy body pathology." *Neurology* 1993; 34:2222–2227.

Good, P., et al. "Neuromelanin-containing neurons of the substantia nigra accumulate iron and aluminum in Parkinson's disease: A LAMMA study." *Brain Res* 1992; 593:3343–3346.

Gorell, J. M., et al. "Occupational exposures to metals as risk factors for Parkinson's disease." *Neurology* 1997b; 48:650–658.

Grandinetti, A., et al. "Prospective study of cigarette smoking and the risk of developing idiopathic Parkinson's disease." *Am J Epidemiol* 1994; 139:1129–1138.

Hubble, J., et al. "Risk factors for Parkinson's disease." *Neurology* 1993; 43:1693–1697.

Hubble, J., et al. "Nocardia species as an etiologic agent in Parkinson's disease: Serological testing in a case-control study." *J Clin Microbiol* 1995; 33:2768–2769.

Janson, A. M., et al. "Differential effects of acute and chronic nicotine treatment on MPTP induced degeneration of nigrostriatal dopamine neurons in the black mouse." *Clin Invest* 1992; 70:232–238.

Jenner, P., and Olanow, C. W. "Oxidative stress and the pathogenesis of Parkinson's disease." *Neurology* 1996; 47:161–170.

Johnson, W. G., Hodge, S. E., and Duvoisin, R. "Twin studies and the genetics of Parkinson's disease—A reappraisal." *Mov Disor* 1990; 5:187–194.

Kondo, K., and Kurland, L. T. "Parkinson's disease: Genetic analysis and evidence of a multfactorial etiology." *Mayo Clinic Proc* 1973; 48:465–474.

Langston, J. W., et al. "Chronic parkinsonism in humans due to a product of meperidine-analog synthesis." *Science* 1983; 219:979–980.

Lazzarini, A. M., et al. "A clinical genetic study of Parkinson's disease: Evidence for dominant transmission." *Neurology* 1994; 44:499–506.

Li, S. C., Schoenberg, B. S., Wang, C. C., et al. "A prevalence survey of Parkinson's disease and other movement disorders in the People's Republic of China." *Arch Neurol* 1985; 42:655–657.

Logroscino, G., et al. "Dietary lipids and antioxidants in Parkinson's disease: A popplulation-based, case-control study." *Ann Neurol* 1996; 39:89–94.

Marjama-Lyons, J., M.D., Parko, K., Singleton, A., et al. "Parkinson's disease in the Navajo." Abstract, Fourteenth International Congress on Parkinson's Disease, Helsinki, Finland, July 2001.

McNaught, K. S. P., et al. "Selective dopaminergic neuronal death with proteinaceous inclusions following impairment of the ubiquitin-proteasome system," Reports from the 54th Annual Meeting of the American Academy of Neurology, April 13–20, 2002. *Neurology* 2002; 58 (supplement 7).

Mjones, H. "Paralysis Agitans. A clinical genetic study." *Act Psychiatr Neurol Scand* 1949; 25:1–195.

Morens, D. M., et al. "The frequency of idiopathic Parkinson's disease by age, ethnic group, and sex in Northern Manhattan, 1988–1993." *Am J Epidemiol* 1996c; 144:198.

Morens, D. M., et al. "Case-control study of idiopathic Parkinson's disease and dietary vitamin E intake." *Neurology* 1996b; 46:1270–1274.

Nelson, L. M., et al. "Incidence of idiopathic Parkinson's disease (PD) in a health maintenance organization (HMO): Variation by age, gender and race/ethnicity." *Neurology* 1997; 48:A334.

Olanow, C. W., et al., "Proteasomal inhibition induces degeneration of dopaminergic neurons with inclusion bodies in the substantia nigra pars compacta of rats," Reports from the 54th Annual Meeting of the American Academy of Neurology, April 13–20, 2002. *Neurology* 2002; 58 (supplement 7).

Ross, G. W., et. al. "Association of coffee and caffeine intake with the risk of Parkinson's disease." *AMA*, May 24, 2000; 283(20):2674–2679.

Schoenberg, B. S., Anderson, D. W., and Haerer, A. F. "Comparison of the prevalence of Parkinson's disease in the biracial population of Copiah County, Mississippi." *Neurology* 1985; 35:841–845.

Tanner, C. M., et al. "Vitamin use and Parkinson's disease." *Ann Neurol* 1988; 233:182.

Tanner, C. M., et al. "Parkinson's disease in twins: An etiologic study," *JAMA* 1999; 281:341–346.

Vieregge, A., et al. "Transdermal nicotine in PD: A randomized, double-blind, placebo-controlled study." *Neurology* 2001; 57:1032–1035.

Wang, S. J., et al. "A door-to-door survey of Parkinson's disease in a Chinese population in Kinmen." *Arch Neurol* 1996; 53:66–71.

Chapter 3

Koller W., *Handbook of Parkinson's Disease.* New York: Marcel Dekker, 1987.

Marjama-Lyons, J., and Koller, W. "Parkinson's disease in diagnosis and symptom management." *Geriatrics* 2001; 56:24–35.

Parkinson, J. *An Essay on the Shaking Palsy.* London: Whittingham and Rowland for Sherwood, Needy and Jones, 1817.

Chapter 4

Gershanik, O., "Parkinson's Disease." In Tolosa, E., Koller, W. C., et. al., *Differential Diagnosis and Treatment of Movement Disorders.* Boston: Butterworth-Heinemann, 1998; pp. 7–25.

Kubler-Ross, E. *On Death and Dying.* New York: Macmillan, 1969.

Marjama-Lyons, J., and Koller, W. "Parkinson's disease: Update in diagnosis and symptom management." *Geriatrics* 2001; 56:24–35.

Piccini, P., et al. "Dopaminergic function in familial Parkinson's disease: A clinical and [F]-dopa PET study." *Ann Neurol* 1997a; 41:222–229.

Chapter 5

Block, G., Liss, C., Reines, S., et al. "Comparison of immediate-release and controlled-release carbidopa/levodopa in Parkinson's disease: A multicenter 5-year study." *Eur Neurol* 1997; 37:23–27.

Corbin, K. B. "Trihexyphenidyl: Evaluation of a new agent in treatment of Parkinson's disease." *JAMA* 1949; 141:377–382.

Cotzias, G. C., Papavasiliou, P. S., and Gellen R. "Modification of parkinsonism: Chronic treatment with L-dopa." *New England Journal of Medicine* 1969; 280:337–345.

Ferrante, C., Perretti, A., Pomati, V., et al. "Botulinum toxin and Parkinson's disease: A new therapeutical approach." Abstract, Parkinsonism and Related Disorders, XIV International Congress on Parkinson's Disease, Helsinki, Finland, August 2001.

Henderson, J. M., Ghinka, J. A., Van Melle, G., et al. "Botulinum toxin A in non-dystonic tremos." *Eur Neruol* 1996; 36:29–35.

Hubble, J., and Berchou, R., *Parkinson's Disease: Medications.* National Parkinson Foundation, Inc., 1501 N.W. Ninth Avenue (Bob Hope Road), Miami, FL 33136-1494.

Kornhuber, J., Weller, M., Schoppmeyer, K., and Riederer, P. "Amantadine and memantadine are NMDA receptor antagonists with neuroprotective properties." *J Neural Transm* 1994; 43(Suppl):S4–S6.

Lees, A. J., et. al. "Ten-year follow-up of three different initial treatments in de-novo PD." *Neurology* 2001; 57:1687–1694.

Marjama-Lyons, J., and Koller, W. "Parkinson's disease: Update in diagnosis and symptom management." *Geriatrics* 2001; 56:24–35.

"New alternative for Parkinson's treatment," *Apples for Health*, vol. 2, no. 21, October 20, 2000.

Olanow, C. W., and Calne, D. "Does selegiline monotherapy in Parkinson's disease act by symptomatic or protective mechanisms?" *Neurology* 1992; 42(Suppl 4):13–26.

Pahwa, R., and Koller, W. C. "Dopamine agonists in the treatment of Parkinson's disease." *Cleve Clin J Med* 1995; 62:212–217.

"Parkinson's drug breakthrough," *BBC News*, October 18, 2000.

Parkinson's Study Group. "Pramipexole vs Levodopa as initial treatment for Parkinson's disease." *JAMA* 2000; 284:1931–1938.

Parkinson Study Group. "The COMT inhibitor entacapone increases on time in Levodopa treated Parkinson's disease patients with motor fluctuations." *Ann Neurol* 1997; 46:747–755.

Parkinson Study Group. Effects of deprenyl on the progression of disability in early Parkinson's disease. *New England Journal of Medicine* 1989; 321:1364–1371.

Rascol, O., Brooks, D. J., Korczyn, A. D., et al. "A five-year study of the incidence of dyskinesia in patients with early Parkinson's disease who were treated with ropinirole or levodopa." *New England Journal of Medicine* 2000; 342(20):1484–1491.

SmithKline Beecham press release, December 14, 1998.

Timberlake, W. H., and Vance, M. A. "Four-year treatment of patients with parkinsonism using amantadine alone or with levodopa." *Ann Neurol* 1978; 3:119–128.

Trosch, R. M., and Pullman, S. L. "Botulinum toxin A injections for the treatment of hand tremors." *Mov Dis* 1994; 9:601–609.

Turski, L., Bressler, K., Retti, K. J., et al. "Protection of substantia nigra from MPP+ neurotoxicity by N-methyl-D-aspartate antagonists." *Nature* 1991; 349:414–418.

Waters, C. H., Kurth, M., Baily, P., et al. "Tolcapone in stable Parkinson's disease: Efficacy and safety of long-term treatment." *Neurology* 1997; 49:665–671.

Chapter 6

Baron, M. S., et al. "Treatment of advanced Parkinson's disease by unilateral posterior GPi pallidotomy: 4-year results of a pilot study." *Mov Disord* 2000; 15:230–237.

Benabid, A. L., et al. "Chronic electrical stimulation of the ventralis intermedius nucleus of the thalamus as a treatment of movement disorders." *J Neurosurg* 1996; 84:203–214.

Burchiel, K. J., et al. "Comparison of pallidal and subthalamic nucleus deep brain stimulation for advanced Parkinson's disease: Results of a randomized, blinded pilot study." *Neurosurg* 1999; 45:1375–1382.

"The Deep Brain Stimulation for Parkinson's Disease Study Group: Deep brain stimulation of the subthalamic nucleus or the pars interna of the globus pallidus in Parkinson's disease." *New England Journal of Medicine* 2001; 345:956–963.

Duma, C. M., et al. "Gamma knife radiosurgery for thalamotomy in Parkinsonian tremor: A five-year experience." *J Neurosurg* 1998; 88:1121–1122.

"Electrical brain stimulation reduces Parkinson's symptoms," *American Academy of Neurology Online,* http://www.aan.com/, November 28, 2001.

Fazzini, E., et al. "Stereotactic pallidotomy for Parkinson's disease: A long-term follow-up of unilateral pallidotomy." *Neurology* 1997; 48:1273–1277.

Freed, C. R., et al. "Transplantation of embryonic dopamine neurons for severe Parkinson's disease." *New England Journal of Medicine* 2001; 344:710–719.

Greene, P. E., et al. "Severe spontaneous dyskinesias: A disabling complication of embryonic dopaminergic tissue implants in a subset of tranplanted patients with advanced Parkinson's disease." *Mov Disord* 1999; 14:904.

Jankovic, J., et al. "Outcome after stereotactic thalamotomy for Parkinsonian, essential and other types of tremor." *Neurosurgery* 1995; 45:1743–1746.

Kelly, P. J., and Gillingham, F. J. "The long-term results of stereo-taxic surgery and L-dopa therapy in patients with Parkinson's disease: A 10 year follow-up study." *J Neurosurg* 1980; 53:322–327.

Krack, P., et. al. "Treatment of tremor in Parkinson's disease by subthalamic nucleus stimulation." *Mov Disord* 1998; 13:907–914.

Lozano, A. M., et al. "Effect of GPI pallidotomy on motor function in Parkinson's disease." *Lancet* 1995; 346:1383–1387.

Medtronic, http://www.medtronic.com, (800) 328-2518

Pahwa, R., et. al. "High frequency stimulation of the globus pallidus for the treatment of Parkinson's disease." *Neurology* 1997; 49:249–253.

Taha, J. M., et. al. "Tremor control after pallidotomy in patients with

Parkinson's disease: Correlation with microelectrode findings." *J Neurosurg* 1997; 86:642–647.

Tasker, R. R. "Deep Brain Stimulation is preferable to thalamotomy for tremor suppression." *Surg Neurol* 1998; 49:145–153.

Vitek, J. L., et. al. "Posteroventral pallidotomy for Parkinson's disease." In Obeso, J. A., ed., *The Basal Ganglia and Surgical Treatment of Parkinson's Disease: Advances in Neurology*, vol. 74. Boston: Lippincott, 1997, pp. 183–198.

Young, R. F. Functional neurosurgery with the Leskell Gamma knife. *Stereotact Funct Neurosurg* 1996; 66:19–23.

Chapter 7

"Advances in treating Parkinson's disease," *Alternative Medicine*, online, May 22, 2000.

Brandabur, Melanie M., and Marjama-Lyons, Jill. "Complementary therapies and Parkinson's disease," National Parkinson Foundation Web site, www.parkinson.org/therapies.htm.

Holistic-online.com—Alternative information, http://www.holistic-online.com/Remedies/Parkinson/pd_diet.htm.

Hubble, Jean Pintar, and Berchou, Richard C. *Parkinson's disease: Medications*, online e-book, National Parkinson's Foundation Web site, www.parkinsons.org.

Larsen, Hans R., "Parkinson's disease: Is victory in sight?" *International Journal of Alternative and Complementary Medicine*, 1997; 15(10):22–24.

Manyam, B. V., and S'anchez-Ramos JR. "Traditional and complementary therapies in Parkinson's disease," *Adv Neurol* 1999; 80:565–574.

Pacchetti, C., et al., "Active Music therapy and Parkinson's disease," *Functional Neurology* 1998; 13(1): 57–67.

Palkhivala, Alison. "Physical therapy could help Parkinson's patients," *WebMD*, May 25, 2001.

"Parkinson's Disease, Herbal and Alternative Medicine." National Parkinson's Foundation fact sheet. http://www.parkinson.org/index.htm.

Rajendran, P., et al. *Neurology* 2000; 54(7 supplement 3):A471–A472. (S80.004). Updated June 2000.

"A rub to treat Parkinson's," *Ivanhoe Newswire*, June 2000.

Toole, T., et al. *NeuroRehabilitation* 2000; 14(3):165–174. Updated October 2000.

Walton-Hadlock, Janice. "Primary Parkinson's disease: The use of Tuina and acupuncture in accord with an evolving hypothesis of its cause from the perspective of Chinese Traditional Medicine—Part 2." *American Journal of Acupuncture* 1999; 27(1/2): 31–49.

Chapter 8

"Advances in treating Parkinson's disease," *Alternative Medicine* magazine online, www.alternativemedicine.com, May 22, 2000.

Atkins, Robert. *Dr. Atkins' Vita-Nutrient Solution*. New York: Simon & Schuster, 1998.

Brandabur, Melanie M., and Marjama-Lyons, Jill. "Complementary therapies and Parkinson's disease," National Parkinson Foundation Web site, www.parkinsons.org/therapies.htm.

Hubble, Jean Pintar, and Berchou, Richard C. *Parkinson's disease: Medications*, online e-book, National Parkinson Foundation Web site, www.parkinson.org.

Holistic-online.com—Alternative information, http://www.holistic-online.com/Remedies/Parkinson/pd_diet.htm.

Larsen, Hans R. "Parkinson's disease: Is victory in sight?" *International Journal of Alternative and Complementary Medicine*; 15(10):22–24.

Last, Walter. "Parkinson's Disease Therapies Protocol." *Life Extension Foundation*, www.lef.org.

Perlmutter, David. *Brainrecovery.Com: Powerful Therapy for Challenging Brain Disorders*. Naples, FL: Perlmutter Publications, 2000.

Riley, David. "Diet and nutrition in Parkinson's disease," Cleveland: Movement Disorders Centre.

Willner, Catherine, "Natural Support for Neurologic Health: A Multiple Pathway Approach." Applied Nutritional Science Reports. June 2001.

Chapter 9

"Age Page on a good night's sleep," *National Institute on Aging* Web site, http://www.nia.nih.gov.

"Age Page on constipation," *National Institute on Aging* Web site, http://www.nia.nih.gov.

"Age Page on depression," *National Institute on Aging* Web site, http://www.nia.nih.gov.

"Age Page on incontinence," *National Institute on Aging* Web site, http://www.nia.nih.gov.

"Ask the pharmacist" column, *Parkinson Report*, Fall 2000 issue, National Parkinson Foundation.

BW HealthWire, August 13, 1998.

Cram, David L. "Freezing in Parkinson's disease: What is it and what can you do about it?" *Parkinson Report*, Fall 2000 issue, National Parkinson Foundation magazine.

"Diphenhudramine linked with delirium in elderly in-patients," *Reuters Health*, December 4, 2001.

Dixon, Bruce. "Walking aids of limited help in Parkinson's," *Reuters Health*, October 3, 2001.

Hyson, H. C., Jog, M. S., and Johnson, A. "Sublingual atropine for sialorrhea secondary to parkinsonism." Abstract, XIV International Congress on Parkinson's Disease, Helsinki, Finland, July 2001.

Independence Dogs Inc., www.independencedogs.com.

Lieberman, A. "Impotence in Parkinson's disease." *CNS Spectrums* 1998; 3:46–52.

Reinberg, Steven. "Parkinson's drugs can cause excessive drowsiness," *Reuters Health*, August 30, 2001.

Slewett, Nathan. "Specially trained dogs help PD patients," *Parkinson Report*, Fall 2000 issue, National Parkinson Foundation magazine.

Zhang, Lin. Proceedings of the American Academy of Neurology's 51st Annual Meeting, April 1999.

Chapter 10

"Choosing a doctor," *National Institute on Aging Age Page*, National Institute on Aging Web site, http://www.nia.nih.gov.

Curry, Pat. "Speaking up is healthy." *HealthScoutNews wire*, October 22, 2001.

Fox, Michael J. Interview with Diane Sawyer. *20/20*, May 17, 2000.

Gibb, W. R. G., and Lees, A. J. "A comparison of clinical and pathological features of young- and old-onset Parkinson's disease." *Neurology* 1988; 38:1402–1406.

Golbe, Lawrence. "Young-onset Parkinson's disease: A clinical review." *Neurology* 1991; 41:168–173.

Hoehn, M. M., and Yarh, M. D. Parkinsonism: Onset, progression and mortality. *Neurology* 1967; 17:427–442.

Kinsley, Michael. "A healthy state of denial," *Guardian*, December 13, 2001.

Rathke, Lisa. "Actor Michael J. Fox addresses second annual disability conference," *Associated Press State & Local Wire*, December 12, 2001.

"Talking with your doctor: A guide for older people," National Institute on Aging Web site, http://www.nia.nih.gov.

Chapter 11

Ahlskog, J. E., and Muenter, M. D. "Frequency of levodopa-related dyskinesia and motor fluctuations as estimated from the cumulative literature." *Mov Disor* 2001; 16:448–458.

Akerud, P., et al. Neuroprotection through delivery of glial cell line-derived neurotrophic factor by neural stem cells in a mouse model of Parkinson's disease." *J Neurosci* 2001; 21:8108–8118.

Bibbiani, Franceso, et. al., "Serotonin 5-HT1A agonist improves motor complications in rodent and primate parkinsonian models," *Neurology* 2001; 57:1829–1834.

Bolanos, J. P., et al. "Nitric oxide-mediated mitochondrial damage: a potential neuroprotective role for glutathione." *Free Radic Biol Med* 1996; 21:995–1001.

Chen, J. F., et al. "Neuroprotection by caffeine A2a adenosine receptor inactivation in a model of Parkinson's disease." *J Neurosci* 2001; 21:RC143.

Choi, D. "Glutamate neurotoxicity and diseases of the nervous system." *Neuron* 1988; 1:623–634.

Dizdar, N., et al. "Treatment of Parkinson's disease with NADH." *Acta Neurol Scand* 1994; 90:345–347.

Fahn, S. "Rotigotine transdermal system (SMP-962) is safe and effective as monotherapy in early Parkinson's disease." Abstract, XIV International Congress on Parkinson's Disease, Helsinki, Finland, July 2001.

Feany, M. B., and Bender, W. W. "A Drosophia model of Parkinson's disease." *Nature* 2000; 404:394–398.

Fox, S. H., et al. "Neural mechanisms underlying peak-dose dyskinesia induced by levodopa and apomorphine are distinct: Evidence from the effects of the alpha-2-adrenoreceptor antagonist, idazoxan." *Mov Disor* 2001; 16:642–650.

Freed, C. R., et al. "Transplantation of embryonic dopamine neurons for severe Parkinson's disease." *New England Journal of Medicine* 2001; 344:710–719.

Gash, D. M., et al. "Functional recovery in parkinsonian monkeys treated with GDNF." *Nature* 1996; 380:252–255.

Grenemayre, T., et al. "Antiparkinsonian effects of ramacemide hydrochloride, a glutamate antagonist, in rodent and primate models of Parkinson's disease." *Ann Neurol* 1994; 35:655–661.

Hoffheimer, L. S. "Congressional hearings held on Parkinson's disease research." *Parkinson Report*, Spring 2000, 18–20 .

Jenner, P., and Olanow, C. W. "Understanding cell death in Parkinson's disease." *Ann Neurol* 1998; 44 (suppl 1):S72–84.

Kitada, T., et al. "Mutations in the parkin gene cause autosomal recessive juvenile parkinsonism." *Nature* 1998; 392:605–608.

Koller, W. C. "Neuroprotection for Parkinson's disease." *Ann Neurol* 1998; 44:S155–159.

Kuno, S., et al. "Selegiline and desmethylselegiline stimulate NGF, BDNF and GDNF synthesis in cultured mouse astrocytes." Abstract, XIV International Congress on Parkinson's Disease, Helsinki, Finland, July 2001.

Minguez, A., et al. "Tranplantation of carotid body cell aggregates in patients with Parkinson's disease: A pilot study." Abstract, XIV International Congress on Parkinson's Disease, Helsinki, Finland, July 2001.

Monte, D., et al. "Glutathione in Parkinson's disease: A link between oxidative stress and mitochondrial damage." *Ann Neurol* 1992; 32:S111–115.

Olanow, C. W., Watts, R., and Koller, W. "An algorithm (decision tree) for the management of Parkinson's disease (2001): Treatment guidelines." *Neurology* 2001; 56:S1–88.

Olanow, C. W., et al. "Neurodegeneration and Parkinson's disease." In J.

Jankovic and E Tolosa, eds., *Parkinson's Disease and Movement Disorders.* Philadelphia, PA: Williams and Wilkins, 1998.

Parkinson Study Group. "Pramipexole vs. Levodopa on the progression of Parkinson's disease." JAMA 2002; 287:1653–1661.

Polymeropoulos, M. H., et al. "Mutation in the alpha-synuclein gene identified in families with Parkinson's disease." *Science* 1997; 276:2045–2047.

Rabey, J. M., and the Rasagiline Study Group. "Rasagiline mesylate, a new MAO-B inhibitor for treatment of Parkinson's disease: A double-blind study as adjunctive therapy to levodopa." Abstract, XIV International Congress on Parkinson's Disease, Helsinki, Finland, July 2001.

Raff, M. C., et al. "Programmed cell death and the control of cell survival: Lessons from the nervous system." *Science* 1993; 262:695–700.

Rajendran, P., et al. "The use of alternative therapies by patients with Parkinson's disease." *Neurology* 2001; 57:790–794.

Rascol, O., et al. "Idazoxan, an alpha-2 antagonist, and L-Dopa-induced dyskinesias in patients with Parkinson's disease." *Mov Disor* 2001; 16:708–713.

Sawada, H., et al. "Dopamine D2-type agonists protect mesencephalic neurons from glutamate toxicity: Mechanisms of neuroprotection treatment against oxidative stress." *Ann Neurol* 1998; 44:110.

Schneider, J. S., et al. "GM1 Ganglioside and Parkinson disease references and summary," of *Science* 1992; 256:843–846, and *Neurology* 1998; 50:1630–1636. http://www.parkinson.org/gm1.htm.

Scott, W. K., et al. "Complete genomic screen in Parkinson's disease: Evidence for multiple genes." *JAMA* 2001; 18:2239–2244.

Shimura, H., et al. "Ubiquitination of a new form of alpha-synuclein by parkin from human brain: Implications for Parkinson's disease." *Science* 2001; 293:263–269.

Steiner, J. P., et al. "Neurotrophic immunophilin ligands stimulate structural and functional recovery in neurodegenerative animal models." *Proc Natl Aca Sci* 1997; 94:2019–2024.

Suuronen, T. P., et al. "Protective effect of L-deprenyl against apoptosis induced by okadaic acid in cultured neuronal cells." *Biochemical Pharmacology* 2000; 59:1589–1595.

Sveinbjornsdottir, S., et al. "Familial aggregation of Parkinson disease in Iceland." *New England Journal of Medicine* 2000; 343:1765.

Tomac, A., et al. "Protection and repair of the nigrostriatal dopmanergic system of GDNF in vivo." *Nature* 1995; 373:355–359.

Turski, L., et al. "Protection of substantia nigra from MPP+ neurotoxicity by NMDA antagonists." *Nature* 1991; 349:414–418.

Watkins, J. C., and Oliverman, H. J. "Agonists and antagonists for excitatory amino acid receptors." *Trends Neurosc* 1987; 10:265–272.

Watts, R. L., Freeman, T. B., Hauser, R. A., et al. "A double-blind, randomized controlled, multi-center clinical trial of the safety and efficacy of stereotaxic intrastriational implantation of fetal porcine ventral mesencephalic tissue (neurocelltm-Parkinson's disease) vs imitation surgery in patients with Parkinson's disease." Abstract, XIV International Congress on Parkinson's Disease, Helsinki, Finland, July 2001.

Watts, R. L., et al. "Stereotaxic intrastriational implantation of retinal pigmented epithelial cells attached to microcarriers in advanced Parkinson's disease patients: A pilot study in six patients." Abstract, XIV International Congress on Parkinson's Disease, Helsinki, Finland, July 2001.

Yansheng, D., et al. "Minocycline prevents nigrostriatal dopmaninergic neurogeneration in the MPTP model of Parkinson's disease." *Proc Natl Aca Sci* 2001; 98:14669.

Zhang, S. C., et al. *Stem Cells Seeded into Brain Become Neural Cells.* http://unisci.com.

Epilogue

Bitzer, Robert. "Belief Comes First." In *Collected Essays of Robert Bitzer,* DeVorss and Company, P.O. Box 550, Marina del Rey, CA 90294, 1990, p. 164.

Daily Word, 1901 NW Blue Parkway, Unity Village, MO 64065-0001.

Shultz, J. Kennedy. *You Are the Power: A Guide to Personal Greatness.* Carlsbad, Calif.: Hay House Inc., 1993.

Index

About the Authors

JILL MARJAMA-LYONS, M.D.

Dr. Jill Marjama-Lyons is a board-certified neurologist with fellowship training in Parkinson's disease. She received her bachelor's degree with honors in psychology from the University of North Carolina at Chapel Hill and her medical degree at S.U.N.Y. Health Sciences Center in Syracuse, New York, having graduated in the upper third of her class. She completed an internship and one year of psychiatry residency at the University of Rochester at Strong Memorial Hospital and then went on to complete her neurology residency at the University of Arizona in Tucson. She then finished a one-year fellowship in Parkinson's disease with Dr. William Koller, an internationally acclaimed Parkinson's disease expert. She spent over four years in private practice neurology in Albuquerque, New Mexico, before becoming medical director of the Parkinson Center at the University of Florida in Jacksonville. She later returned to New Mexico to write, teach, and learn from the Navajo people. Dr. Jill has written numerous articles, given over one hundred lectures, served on national advisory panels, and received awards for outstanding achievement in her field. She firmly believes in holistic treatment of Parkinson's disease and practices what she preaches. She earned her brown belt in shotokan karate, practices yoga and t'ai chi along with other exercise, meditates, prays, and takes antioxidants. She is involved in clinical research in traditional and alternative therapies for Parkinson's disease and encourages her patients to consider adding alternative therapies to conventional medicines for the treatment of PD. You can visit her on the Web at http://www.docjill.com.

MARY J. SHOMON

Mary Shomon, a graduate of Georgetown University in Washington, D.C., is a writer on health and wellness issues, a patient advocate, and a health communications consultant. She is the author of the bestselling book *Living Well with Hypothyroidism: What Your Doctor Doesn't Tell You . . . That You Need to Know* (HarperCollins, 2000), which was voted one of Amazon's top fifty health bestsellers for 2000 and 2001. The *Los Angeles Times* has said of this book, which went into twelve printings in less than two years after publication, "Shomon . . . challenges patients and their doctors to look deeper and try harder to resolve the complicated symptoms." Mary is also the author of *Living Well with Autoimmune Disease* (HarperCollins, 2002). She is founder of the popular Web sites http://www.thyroid-info.com and http://thyroid.about.com, and her writing and patient advocacy work combining educational information on both conventional and alternative therapies has been featured in national media such as ABC News, the *New York Times*, the *Houston Chronicle*, the Associated Press, *Women's World, Ladies' Home Journal*, CBS Radio, NBC Radio, the Canadian Broadcasting Company (CBC), and dozens of other magazines, radio networks, and television stations. Mary practices yoga and t'ai chi and regularly receives acupuncture, herbal remedies, and Reiki treatments for her own chronic autoimmune disease. You can visit her on the Web at http://www.thyroid-info.com.

WHAT YOUR DOCTOR MAY *NOT* TELL YOU ABOUT FIBROMYALGIA

The Revolutionary Treatment That Can Reverse the Disease
by R. Paul St. Amand, M.D., and Claudia Craig Marek

In this innovative book, Dr. St. Amand, the country's foremost expert on this subject and a former sufferer of fibromyalgia, presents his amazing discoveries based on forty years of research. This book offers the first effective protocol for reversing fibromyalgia: a program that uses guaifenesin, an inexpensive, proven-safe medication available from your doctor. This is the definitive guide to this troubling, often misdiagnosed disease.

"Groundbreaking. . . . Dr. St. Amand's research will permit fibromyalgia to become merely a memory."
— Dr. John Willems, M.D., head, Division of Obstetrics and Gynecology, Scripps Clinic

WHAT YOUR DOCTOR MAY *NOT* TELL YOU ABOUT KNEE PAIN AND SURGERY

Learn the Truth about MRIs and Common Misdiagnoses—
and Avoid Unnecessary Surgery
by Ronald P. Grelsamer, M.D.

Why do MRIs sometimes lead to misdiagnosed knee conditions? Why are millions of people receiving unnecessary knee surgery? In this clear, candid book, noted orthopedic surgeon Dr. Ronald P. Grelsamer exposes the potential dangers of misread MRIs and explains why surgery is often not required to alleviate many types of knee pain. Ideal for the millions of knee-pain sufferers of all ages who are looking for solutions other than surgery, this guide equips you with expert advice on relieving pain for virtually every knee condition, including arthritis, runner's knee, torn ligaments and cartilage, tendinitis, and more.

"Finally, a knee book that tells it like it is."

—Lewis Maharam, M.D., FACSM, president,
Greater New York Regional Chapter,
American College of Sports Medicine

WHAT YOUR DOCTOR MAY *NOT* TELL YOU ABOUT MIGRAINES

The Breakthrough Program That Can Help End Your Pain
by Alexander Mauskop, M.D., and Barry Fox, Ph.D.

Some twenty-five million Americans suffer from excruciating headaches that can last for hours or even days. Current treatments and prescription drugs fail to help millions of these patients. But now there's a safe, all-natural "triple therapy" program that *can* relieve the pain—and often even prevent recurrences—of migraines. A combination of three easy-to-find, over-the-counter supplements, this scientifically proven remedy was developed by one of the nation's leading migraine experts and has already helped thousands.

"Natural, safe, and very effective . . . an exciting new approach . . . the solution millions of migraineurs have been waiting for."

—Allen Montgomery, president,
The American Nutraceutical Association